Radiographic Processing & Quality Control

Radiographic Processing & Quality Control

William E. J. McKinney

E. I. Du Pont de Nemours & Co., Inc.
Chestnut Run Laboratories
Customer Technology Center
Wilmington, Delaware

J. B. Lippincott Company

Philadelphia

London   Mexico City   New York   St. Louis   São Paulo   Sydney

Acquisitions Editor: Lisa A. Biello
Manuscript Editor: Helen Ewan
Indexer: Nancy Newman
Design Coordinator: Paul Fry
Production Manager: Kathleen P. Dunn
Production Coordinator: Fred D. Wood, IV
Cover Design: Paul Fry
Compositor: Maryland Composition Company, Inc.
Printer/Binder: Murray Printing Company

1   3   5   6   4   2

Library of Congress Cataloging-in-Publication Data

McKinney, William E. J.
    Radiographic processing and quality control / William E. J. McKinney.
        p.   cm.
    Bibliography: p.
    Includes index.
    ISBN 0-397-50902-2
    1. Radiography, Medical—Processing.   2. Radiography, Medical—Quality
control.   I. Title.
RC78.M325   1988
616.07′7572—dc 19   87-36460
                                                                             CIP

Preface

There is much that needs to be set forth and set straight about the importance of processing in the formation of the useful visible image. Some training programs presented by various companies have concentrated only on electromechanics: how the processor works and how to fix it. Few courses offer any insight into the chemical reactions that occur during processing. For almost twenty years, the Du Pont Processing School trained many thousands in electromechanics, chemistry, sensitometry, and quality control. It favored no particular type of processor, film, or chemistry.

Radiographic Processing and Quality Control is a result of that educational program. It provides the first modern, in-depth review of all of the aspects of processing, processors, and quality control.

A complete reference text for the small doctor's office and the university medical center must take a broad approach. Mechanics and electricity are discussed so that anyone interested in working with processors can do so. More important, however, the mechanics and electricians who are unfamiliar with processors can gain insight. Chemistry is included to support the work of quality control staff, technologists, physicists, chief technologists, and instructors. Quality control is intended to be introductory to some and will encourage and motivate others to seek higher levels of understanding and achievement.

Some sections may seem repetitious, but this is by design. As an educational text, each section is complete. As a reference text, the same subject is discussed in different sections so that the reader does not have to search through various sections.

For the most part, the text is composed of short declarative sentences, designed to meet the need of providing maximum information without excess words. It will, perhaps, seem stunted, but it is easier to read than other styles.

Within these pages are years of experience. Hopefully, basic concepts will emerge. For instance, one of my favorite sayings is, "Don't fix the processor if it is not the source of the problem." If the chemistry is at fault, fix it. If the exposure technique is at fault, fix it. Of course, the problem is that one must know all of the cause and effect relationships. Included herein is information that both supports and takes the reader far beyond the information supplied in processor manuals and general radiographic technology texts.

The purpose of *Radiographic Processing and Quality Control* is to foster in medical radiography better diagnostic quality, consistent diagnostic quality, and the best possible medicine at the least possible cost to the patient.

William E. J. McKinney

Contents

Introduction

Most radiographers (radiologic technologists, radiographic technologists, registered technologists, technologists) are highly skilled, motivated, and generally interested in the challenges of creating an image on film. Much training goes into being able to select the correct exposure. However, the "image" or "exposure" is useless until it is developed. This image is called a *latent image*. It is through the chemical process called development that the hidden, latent image is transformed into the useful *visible image*. For any radiographer, to know only about latent image formation and not visible image formation is to know only half of the technology called radiography. Radiographers must be knowledgeable and skilled in both areas to control the efficiency, economics, and quality for which they are responsible.

The basic steps in processing are *development* (converts latent image into visible image), *fixation* (stops development and removes all remaining undeveloped crystals and unexposed crystals), *washing* (removes fixer to ensure archival quality), and *drying*. All of the chemical reaction steps are controlled by elements of time (immersion time in solution), temperature (of the solution), and activity (replenishment, agitation, moisture, etc.). These functions are served by various systems such as transport (time factor), temperature control, replenishment, circulation/filtration (agitation, uniformity of chemicals), dryer, and electrical systems. These six electromechanical systems (electricity-powered mechanical devices) constitute the *processor* (manual or automatic). In processing, there are seven systems: the six supporting electromechanical processor systems are based on the needs of the seventh system, which is chemistry (developer, fixer, and wash). While the developer has its own time/temperature/activity relationship, so do the fixer and the wash. It is a fact that one of the controlling factors of the developer is the fixer; if the fixer is not washed out properly, the film is damaged. Moreover, this is why there is a general transport system for all stages rather than a "developer transport system," "fixer transport system," and so on.

How does one know if the "processor" is working right? This really means, how does one know if processing is correct? Will it produce a good radiograph? If a technically accurate "exposure" (exposed radiograph with a latent image) is put into a processor, will it come out okay? Will it be free of artifacts and have the correct density and contrast? What if there is a question about the exposure technique and whether it is really optimal? Then, when the visible film is read, what if the question is raised about whether the quality achieved is the result of bad exposure, bad processing, or both? The answer to all of these questions, which are quite common in radiography, is in two parts. *First, there is no value greater than correct exposure with full development.* Overexposure with underdevelopment or vice versa is hazardous, inappropriate, and inefficient. The processing completes what the exposure started. It cannot add information. *Second, the goal of the radiographer's efforts is to produce a useful visible image.* This image may be measured in terms of its density levels and contrast. These are called sensitometric values. Thus, to monitor and control processing and the total visible image production, sensitometry is used. Most people simply call it *quality control. Sensitometry* may be defined as the quantitative measure of the film's response to exposure and development. The total value of the visible image is the result of exposure *and* development. To know only how to make exposures is to know only half of the technology required.

It is the intention of *Radiographic Processing and Quality Control* to develop the other half of the technologist's skills: visible image formation. This book is comprehensive, offering basic information and some guidance in procedures such as processor maintenance schedules, testing chemicals, and artifact interpretation. It should be a source of learning and a ready reference for daily operation.

Radiographic Processing & Quality Control

Chapter 1

Darkroom/Processing Areas

Principle

The radiographic darkroom is two things: a scientific laboratory and a *dark* room. A darkroom—a room where the lighting is of very low level and special light filters are used—must be constantly inspected to ensure that it is indeed dark. The reason is that radiographic film is sensitive to light, which will expose it and turn it black after processing. Radiographic (x-ray) film can be affected by heat, light, humidity, static electricity, pressure, chemical fumes, and radiation. Since so many things can alter radiographic film, the darkroom must be considered a scientific laboratory. As in any laboratory, certain dictates of common sense are required to establish and maintain a desired level of quality. All variables that can alter the scientific processes within the darkroom must be found and eliminated. A routine system of checking for these variables must be established.

To reinforce the concept of the darkroom as a scientific laboratory that exists in the dark, consider just two points. First, radiography strives to make diagnostic-quality radiographs. The most common cause of unsatisfactory radiographs is fog. Fog is noninformational density, or blackness from silver deposits that occur in the wrong place, masking the visibility of detail. As mentioned above, many energy levels cause radiographic film to become exposed and, after processing, to become black. Once radiation exposure has been made, the radiographic film becomes at least twice as sensitive to all energy levels, and thus extreme care is required in working within the darkroom laboratory. Second, the darkroom laboratory exists because a very precise manner of processing is required to change the image formed by the exposure (the latent image) into the useful visible image. Processing is an exact science based on a scientific principle called the time/temperature method of processing. This time/temperature principle is based on a controlled level of chemical activity, all aspects of which are controlled by the darkroom technician or radiographer. Correct processing is vital to radiography and must be performed with complete precision.

The darkroom laboratory must admit no white light and should meet all of the requirements and have all of the equipment of a laboratory. Most laboratories are well-ventilated, well-organized, clean, pleasant, and safe places to work. This then should be a starting point for consideration of a darkroom design.

Darkroom Design

Function

The darkroom has special lighting to permit film to be removed from a storage box, loaded into an exposure device (cassette), unloaded, and processed. In a centralized location, it becomes the heart of a radiographic department because all areas and specialty exposure rooms must bring their cassettes to the darkroom for reloading and processing the film. As an old saying goes, "Radiography begins and ends in the darkroom."

The darkroom, as a hub of production, must be designed and worked for the greatest efficiency. Darkroom personnel (technicians) should be able to do most of their work taking very few steps in the unloading, reloading, and processing of film. The greatest inefficiency occurs when the technicians can unload films faster than an automatic processor can accept them. To remedy this, two processors may be installed instead of one to double the film-feeding rate. The second common bottleneck occurs if technologists and/ or students all work in the darkroom rather than one or two designated people (called darkroom technicians). The crowding is inefficient, and there is a general lack of quality in handling films.

Design

The darkroom should be a pleasant, efficient place to work. It should be designed by someone who understands its importance to the department's economy and efficiency.

Entrances in older institutions often were bulky mazes or double doors designed to trap white light or to ensure that it could not enter the darkroom. Modern devices are more versatile, save space, and perhaps are even more efficient. These include the revolving door, which is a tube, and a Beta door. The revolving door has an inner tube with a single large opening; the outer tube has an opening in the darkroom and the light room. To enter, rotate the inner tube until its opening lines up with the outer tube opening. Step in, and rotate the inner tube to the rear exit. Beta doors are a box device with shutters at the entrance and exit. As you approach the door, you must step on a ramp that activates a switch, which pulls open the two halves of the door. Once you are inside the box, the entrance door closes and the exit door opens. Step out, and the exit door recloses. If there is a power failure, the Beta door opens automatically or can be manually opened. In these two systems, locks and alarms are not needed. With conventional darkroom doors, it is desirable to hook an interlock mechanism to the door to prevent its being opened if the film bin is open. A communication system (grill, intercom, phone, etc.) is also advised. Whenever a locking device is used, gaining entry may be a problem if something happens to the darkroom technician or if a fire starts. All darkrooms must have a second emergency exit, possibly a simple kick-out panel. However, it must be designed so that someone can get through it in either direction.

Work flow should require the fewest physical steps or procedures to ensure maximum efficiency. In manual processing, when this operation is performed totally inside the darkroom it is imperative that the wet processing area be as far from the dry area (film storage, cassette loading, etc.) as possible to prevent cross-contamination. It is as if the darkroom were two separate rooms designed for two different functions: a dry area for film loading and a wet area for processing. In addition, space is needed for storage of hangers, the devices used for holding the film for processing. For automatic processing, it is usual and most desirable to place only the feed tray or entrance of the processor in the darkroom. The bulk of the unit is on the other side of the wall in the light source. Figure 1-1 shows examples of darkroom designs and work-flow diagrams.

Ventilation is very important in the darkroom to remove chemical fumes and excess humidity and to aid air-conditioning. If the darkroom environment is good for the technicians it will be good for the film, and vice versa. A typical darkroom should have a ventilator in the lower portion of the entrance door or in the wall near the floor. At the opposite end of the room, there should be an exhaust fan in the ceiling. Fresh air should flow past the worker, then move on past processing areas to the exhaust. There should not be any pockets of stale air or fumes.

Color selection is generally a personal choice, since a wide selection is available. However, pastels and light colors are preferred because they increase reflectance of available light. Enamels or epoxy paints that are easy to clean should be used, but a matte finish is required. A high-gloss surface will reflect light leaks and may cause problems. Even though the surface is easy to clean, someone has to clean it regularly—it will not clean itself.

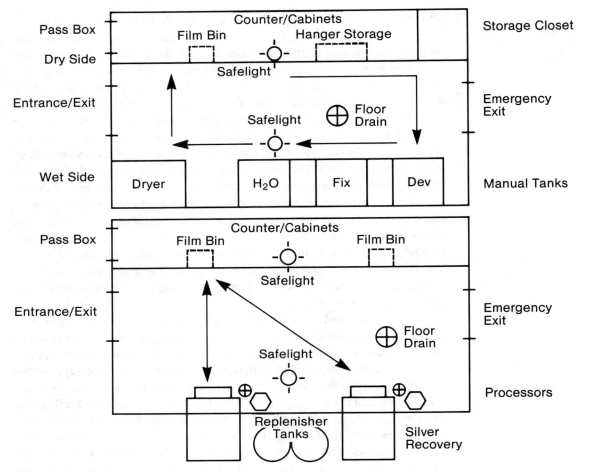

Fig. 1-1.   Darkroom Designs.

Radiation protection is only a problem if one or more of the darkroom walls is common to a radiographic exposure room. In that case, it must be tested initially and regularly thereafter to ensure that stray radiation is not penetrating the darkroom. The easiest test is to place a penny on a pouch (made of black plastic) of x-ray film and place this device on a wall. The penny is next to the wall. If radiation comes through the wall, the penny will act as a filter and its image will be seen on the processed film. Put up several test units in different places and allow them to remain in place for a month. Another easy test is to use a spare personal radiation monitoring device (film badge) and tape it to the wall or simply issue it to the darkroom technician to wear. If abnormal radiation levels are suspected or found, they must be corrected immediately. Keep records of all tests, even when negative.

Lighting in the darkroom should be of three different types: white light, bright safelight, and normal safelight. White light is required when cleaning up the darkroom, working on cassettes, etc. The lighting should be at least at normal hospital levels (approximately one 2′ × 4′ by 4 tube bank, 500-W fluorescent unit, or equivalent per 0.74 m² [8 ft²]). Bright safelights are special devices. They are used when brighter than normal safelighting is needed, such as when looking for special films or emulsion numbers, when training personnel, or when doing duplication or other special work. The most common type is a sodium vapor light that gives off an orange-yellow glow like streetlights. These lights are expensive and do not turn on and off rapidly. The light intensity is adjustable by using shutters or doors. For similar intensity but a less expensive and a more versatile alternative, use a Kodak Mor-Lite filter in a standard fixture with a 7½- to 15-W bulb. Both of these units must be used indirectly, such as by bouncing the light off a surface. They are usually hung from the ceiling but facing upward. Not as bright is the newer Kodak GBX all-purpose filter, which is more red. Normal safelights are the Kodak Wratten Series 6B, which has a brownish color. It should have a 7½- to 15-W frosted light bulb and be mounted 1.22 m (4 ft) above the work surface, facing downward. Often times, too many safelights are used or they are too close to the work surface, resulting in exposure to the film. Safelights mounted over a processor feed tray should be connected to the processor so that they turn off when the film is fed into the sensor switch. Some special films, which are generally called new-modality films (for computerized tomography, ultrasound, nuclear medicine, magnetic resonance imaging, and lasers), are based on cine emulsion technology and are sensitive to red light and thus require a dark green filter or no lights at all. The dark green filter is very dark. When working in the darkroom, allow your eyes to adjust to the low level of light and inspect for white leaks. All lights should have separate switches. The white light switch must have a lock and/or a cover to prevent accidental activation.

Safelights are not safe until proven safe through a simple test. A light may become unsafe as a result of cracks in the dyed gelatin layer, pin holes, or use of a bulb with the wrong wattage. Safelights should be checked at least quarterly. Test each light individually with all others turned off, then test with all lighted to measure the total effect. Testing requires a sensitized film. Load a cassette and expose it to radiation at about 70 kVp, 2 mAs, 1.02 m (40 inches), on the tabletop to produce a noticeable but very light optical density (OD) of 0.30 to 0.50 on the film when processed. In the darkroom, with all lights off, place the exposed film under the light to be tested, cover all but 2.54 cm (1 inch) of the film with a piece of cardboard (cassette, black film, etc.), and turn the light on. After 10 seconds, move the cover back to expose another 2.54 cm (1 inch). When the entire film length has been exposed except the last 2.54 cm (1 inch), turn off the safelight and process the film. Look at the processed film on a view box. The first exposed strip received the longest safelight exposure, the last strip the least. Label the strips by total time of exposure. Where there is an increase in density above the base plus fog (B + F) level (the first step) determines the maximum amount of time an exposed film can be placed under that one, single safelight before it becomes fogged by the secondary exposure of the safelight. This should be 40 seconds or more but will vary with film products and circumstances such as a damaged filter. Steps should be taken to avoid safelight fog.

Maintenance procedures involve keeping the darkroom dark (checking for and eliminating light leaks as they occur) and clean. At the beginning of each shift or workday, all horizontal planes should be wiped off with a damp rag. The walls should be wiped down weekly. The area should be straightened up and organized for the busy day ahead. If supplies are needed, they should be obtained. Make sure the floor is clean and dry. Inspect the silver recovery device, processor, replenishment tanks, and drains for leaks and proper function. After all of the above is done with the white light on and the inspection has been recorded on a chart or in a book, turn off the lights, allow your eyes to adjust, and inspect for light leaks. Turn on each safelight and look at it to detect cracks, scratches, etc. Smoking and eating should be prohibited in the darkroom.

Static electricity occurs in nonconductive material such as plastic (film base, synthetic-fiber clothing) and builds up until it reaches a potential to allow a rapid discharge in the form of a spark. Film is made of nonconductive base (a good static producer) and emulsion layers on each side. The emulsion layer contains gelatin that is a semiconductor and a mild static producer. Static generated in the base as the film is banged around inside the cassette can escape only through the gelatin layers, which also contain the recording media (silver halide crystals). Thus the discharge is recorded as a pile of silver in the form of a tree, a crown, or smudge static markings (see Chapter 9, Figs. 9-9 and 9-10). To prevent the rapid discharge (the spark), it is important to provide as many avenues as possible for the electricity to dissipate (bleed off) gradually. The exposure table or holder must be grounded, as must the passbox (which cannot be lined with rubber or plastic) and the darkroom work bench. The technician should be encouraged to wear leather-soled shoes rather than rubber and to wear natural-fiber clothing rather than synthetic (plastic, nylon, polyester, etc.) to reduce the sources of static electricity. In addition, the relative humidity in the darkroom should be 40 to 60% at all times. If the humidity is too low, a humidifier may be installed. Another alternative is to use an ion generator, which will also provide multiple paths for the static electricity to bleed off and prevent a rapid discharge.

Ambient conditions in a darkroom should be about 20°C (70°F) throughout the workday. During downtime the temperature may be lower. Temperature should never exceed 24°C (75°F) at any time. Humidity should always range between 40 and 60%, and there should be continuous ventilation to prevent fumes from accumulating. Unfortunately, some darkrooms start the day cool and dry and end up hot and humid. This is to be avoided for the job satisfaction of the technician and to protect the film from artifacts. If the technician is perspiring and the moisture causes the film to be repeated, this in turn costs the hospital money as a result of inefficiency and costs the patient additional radiation and trauma. Be sure to inspect and record the conditions daily around the clock and to correct any problems found. Humidity is measured with a psychrometer. A manual sling psychrometer is inexpensive and easy to use.

Pass boxes allow cassettes to be passed from the darkroom into an exposure room and back again. They must be safe against radiation to protect the film sitting in the pass box and the darkroom technician on the opposite side of the exposure room wall. They must be grounded to help prevent discharge of static electricity. Make sure it is understood which side contains the unexposed cassettes (right side—darkroom; left side—exposure room) and which side contains the exposed cassettes. Confusing these two results in double exposures and inefficiency.

Storage is required in the form of a broom closet, locker, and/or a drawer to contain cleaning supplies, general tools such as scissors and pens, and personal items. If mops, sponges, rags, and a bucket are handy in the darkroom, it is easy for the technician to perform routine maintenance and to handle emergencies. Work tools and personal items must never be carelessly left on a work counter because they might result in damage to a film.

The floor should have a large centrally located drain to handle spills and to facilitate cleanup. The flooring material must be moisture resistant, easy to clean, and of a light color. Where processors drain into the floor, the opening should be loosely sealed with scrap film to control noise and humidity. A plumber can also connect the drain using an open T fitting, which accomplishes the same job. A tray made of plastic or stainless steel should be placed beneath the silver recovery units and replenishment tanks to prevent floor damage. If rubber mats are used to reduce technicians' fatigue, then additional antistatic grounding strips should be placed along the front edge of the work counter to bleed static from the technician. A better floor cover is wooden egg-crate flooring.

Safety becomes an important issue because the darkroom technician is working in a low light (blind) environment or may actually be blind. Great care is needed to ensure that everything is clean and put away in assigned places and that lines of communication are established. A loose screw or sharp edge found by a blind technician should be reported and immediately repaired. In addition, a sighted supervisor or sighted technician should purposely inspect everything about once a week. Keep a record book of all activity. Inspect for radiation protection and the grounding of all work surfaces and equipment including safelights. Restrict access to the area. Supervisors should establish emergency procedures in the event of fire or technician health problems. The darkroom is a vital area, and it is unique because it functions in the dark—which is not as safe as a well-lighted environment.

Drain pipe may be of cast iron or plastic (polyvinylchloride [PVC]). Copper and copper-bearing metals must not be used because the acid fixer will eat them away. Glass drains are expensive and not necessary. PVC pipes may not meet some local codes. The floor drain must be able to handle 2.5 times the maximum outflow of the processor when all drains are open. This is about 38 L/minute (10 gallons/minute). Because these drains constantly flow with water, they must be dedicated to processors and/or manual tanks only. Slope must be greater than minimal. A clean-out trap should be provided. Water must be run whenever chemicals are drained to help keep the drains open. Fixer from a silver recovery unit should be placed in a drain separate from the main drain, if possible and practical. One type of recovery unit uses metallic displacement buckets or cartridges with steel wool. As the steel wool breaks down, particles of iron oxide flush into the drain. If developer hydroxide is in the drain, the iron reacts to form ferris hydroxide, a sticky fiber that clogs the drain. Drains can be cleaned periodically with commercial-grade acid drain cleaners. If a drain totally clogs, have a plumber clean it out, not just "rod" it, which clears only a small hole that easily reclogs.

Training Darkroom Personnel

The primary objective of the darkroom technician and, therefore, of his or her training is the unloading of the exposed film from the cassette. This film is at least twice as sensitive to further exposure, and it represents a financial investment by the hospital and a health investment by the patient in terms of trauma and absorbed radiation dose. It is more difficult to remove the exposed film from the cassette than it is to load a fresh film into a cassette. The technician should be instructed how to unload a cassette properly and then to reload it, not the other way. Actually, it is advisable not to reload cassettes until needed. The film bin, white light, door closure, safelights, pass boxes, and cleanliness are the next aspects of training.

In feeding the film into an automatic processor, the film is lined up along a side edge (rail) and pushed in by placing the fingers at the back edge of the film. Fingers must never be placed on top of the film.

The technician should be instructed not to wear clothing made of synthetic fibers (manmade = plastic) garments which can produce static electricity. Since restricting the choice of clothing may prove unpractical or economically unacceptable, an alternative is to have the technician wear a natural fiber (cotton) smock and ensure proper grounding and darkroom humidity levels.

Larger film should be handled with two hands to avoid kinks and should always be placed on the feed tray, not thrown at it. Film should be placed in cassettes, not slid in.

A lined drawer or box should be available to store films when unloading occurs faster than the processor feed rate. The darkroom technician should be taught how to place new boxes of film in the film bin and how to estimate the amount remaining so that the film supply is not depleted. Packs of film should have their outer wrappers folded down to cover sharp box edges. If the film used has a plastic bag, the bag can be left upright to provide a little extra protection against fogging due to white light. The bag will not interfere with the selection and removal of a film. The technician must be advised about care in the use of hand creams and lotions, and generally to wash and dry hands frequently during the day. Smoking and eating in the darkroom must be prohibited.

Manual Processing Tanks

Manual processing tanks are generally about 0.9 to 2.5 m (3 to 8 ft) long by 0.6 m (2 ft) wide and consist of a large stainless steel tank outer shell. Inside this shell are placed individual 18.9- to 37.9-L (5 to 10 gallon) tanks for each of the chemicals, in sequence: developer, short stop, fixer, hypo eliminator, and wash. The dryer is a separate cabinet. The outer tank forms the wash tank and also a water jacket to heat the other chemicals. These tanks should be as far from the cassette unloading and film bin as possible to ensure that chemicals do not damage the film or screens. With the advent and acceptance of automatic processors, manual tanks (also called hand tanks or deep tanks) were left in the darkroom in case of processor failure. Most institutions have found the processor sufficiently reliable and have never used the manual tanks, which in that case should be removed and sold to make more space. If the backup concept is still desired, consider that the replenishment tanks can be used as manual tanks since they are at 20°C (70°F). The only problem is whether or not the light area, where the tanks are located, can be made into a darkroom.

If manual tanks are retained, they must be thoroughly cleaned and left completely dry. Nothing should be stored within them or on top of them. If they are used occasionally, top up the solution level, stir to mix the chemicals, clean and replace the lid after each use, and drain and replace the chemicals monthly.

Automatic Processors

Automatic processors are of three basic sizes: floor, intermediate, and tabletop. They may be installed as part of the standard darkroom or as part of a centralized or dispersed daylight system. The darkroom installation may be one of three methods: totally inside, the bulk inside, or the bulk outside.

Location of the processor is often dictated by the size of the area, which is unfortunate because the area should be custom designed for the processor and the work at hand to achieve the greatest efficiency. Placing a tabletop or other processor totally inside the darkroom offers the least advantage because it consumes space and generates noise and heat.

The heat factor must be compensated for by increased ventilation and/

or air-conditioning. The bulk-inside installation has the same disadvantage as totally inside, except the exit is through the wall so that films are delivered to the lighted area. In the case of totally inside, the films must be taken outside. However, one advantage in both of these installations is the ability to work on a jammed processor in the dark and perhaps to salvage some films. This is balanced by the disadvantage that you cannot turn on white lights or service the processor without stopping or interfering with the darkroom operation. Thus there are many negative points that suggest these are the least desirable installations. Usually only the feed tray is found within the darkroom, with the bulk outside in the lighted area. The obvious disadvantage is that it is difficult to salvage films in a lighted area. The remedy is to design the lighted area so it can be made dark by closing doors or drawing special window shades.

Processor utilities must be specified. The exact amount and type of water, drain, electrical service, exhaust, and heat service are specified in the installation instructions for each processor and must be considered when designing a darkroom. To simply plug in a processor to an unknown utility will result in problems. Normally all utilities are in the darkroom and attach to the processor under the feed tray. Although this is acceptable for electricity and water input, it may not be for the waste drain or dryer exhaust. The waste drain may be located in the lighted area. In the darkroom, the waste drain must have a free fall so that if the drain clogs it will not back up into the processor. However, installation to accomplish this can be done in several ways to eliminate the noise, splash, and humidity associated with a typical open drain. The dryer exhaust produces a lot of heat, several thousand BTUs per hour, in the darkroom as it passes through. The exhaust duct may be in the lighted area or may pass out the bottom of the processor into the exhaust system for the floor below. In any case, there must be an exhaust system to the outside of the building; exhausted air cannot enter the air-conditioning system.

A processor should never be against a wall, but if it is, place it on a dolly or skid to facilitate service. The minimum space on all sides of a processor should be 60 cm (24 inches). Service cannot be conducted in less space.

Film Identifiers

Film identifiers are very important but are most often installed and forgotten. They may consist of a simple box that flashes light through a card to expose the film to identify it. They might be more elaborate and include the date and time of exposure. In all cases, the placement of the unit requires considerable thought. Make certain it is mounted squarely and is properly grounded to prevent static and shocks. Establish a quality control program that includes checking the image quality (brightness, sharpness, alignment) and mechanical integrity. Mechanically, make certain screws do not work free or that switches become loose. Clean the unit daily and keep records of your activity. This simple device needs a basic maintenance program. Two common problems are light leaks and static electrical discharge.

Daylight and Cassetteless Radiography

There are systems that reduce or eliminate the need for a conventional darkroom. Their advantages include reduced film handling, better quality, improved personnel utilization, and increased space. In a daylight system, the film is loaded into a cassette, exposed, unloaded, and then processed— all in white light or special lighting. One daylight system, the 3M Company's Hi-Lite system, turned an exposure room into a bright lighted darkroom. In the Du Pont Daylight system, all of the operations are mechanical. Film dispensers load special cassettes that are unloaded directly into processors after exposure. Processors can be placed anywhere, producing a decentralized or dispersion processing system. Each technologist loads, exposes, and unloads (processes) films right in or next to the exposure room. Cassettes remain in the exposure room. All of a patient's films will be out of one processor and in the sequence taken.

A modern version of daylight systems is found in centralized daylight units that unload cassettes, identify the film, process the film, and reload the cassette. Many different film sizes and types can be dispersed from one unit.

Cassetteless radiography is primarily made by the x-ray generator companies who build film dispensers into the exposure tables, such as the Picker Rapido Table. Magazines of various sizes are loaded in a conventional darkroom just like a serial changer magazine (Schonander, Puck, Sanchez-Perez), which is another form of cassetteless radiography. The magazine is placed in the table unit. The technologist selects the film which is placed into position. The exposure is made, and the film is ejected. The film usually travels down a conveyor to the foot of the table, where it is fed directly into a processor. This form of cassetteless radiography is not very common. A very common form often overlooked is the automatic chest changer. These units may feed the exposed film directly to a processor or to a magazine that is removed to a conventional darkroom for processing.

Light-Room Design

General Conditions

The light-room area, outside the darkroom, is very important and requires design thought. Processing chemicals should be stored in this area. Films are sorted and reviewed in this area. It is a busy area with people moving about. If repair work must be performed on the processor or if chemicals must be added to the replenishment tanks, then the area must be secured for the safety of the workers and all others. Processor tops must not be used as countertops. Countertops on hinges may be mounted over processors, replenishment tanks, or even between processors. They are easily moved away for service.

View Box Quality Control

The view box is perhaps the single major cause of poor-diagnostic-quality films because it has a direct effect on radiographic contrast (the sum of subject contrast, film contrast, technique, and processing). Contrast enhances the visibility of detail and allows us to see information. View boxes are a light source that should be consistent.

Testing a view box requires a light meter that has an exposure value (EV) scale. EV is a measure of total exposure, so f-stop, aperture, and speed functions do not require consideration. Set the meter to ASA 100, make certain the lens is uncovered for direct reading (the diffuser is off or open), place the meter on the lighted view box, and read the EV in several places. An EV of 13 means there are 5882 lumens/m^2 (500 foot-candles) of power from the view box. All units of the view box should have equal output. If one section has an EV of 14, then twice the light is being emitted, which will make all of the films look too light. If EV 12 is found, then there is only half the light, and all films (the same ones) on that section will appear too dark. If any one portion of a view box is in error, replace all the bulbs. Make certain that all the view boxes in one room are matched. If one bulb burns out, replace all the bulbs. Fluorescent bulbs deteriorate very slowly. The quality control technologist should have the best or standard view box, with all others matched to it.

Cleaning the exterior of the view box daily will remove crayon marks, which could interfere with diagnosis. Once every quarter, the view box should be disassembled and completely cleaned. Dust accumulation can reduce the light output at a rate of about 10% per year. Any rusty metal should be cleaned, primed, and painted with a high-gloss enamel. The exterior surface will become contaminated and stained by tobacco smoke, so smoking should be prohibited or cleaning increased to compensate. Cleaning is performed with a soft rag and liquid glass cleaner or mild soap.

The recommendation for view boxes is EV 13, at ASA 100, for light intensity at the view-box surface and uniform color. X-ray film has a blue tint in the base to reduce eye fatigue. However, certain color combinations can increase or decrease the apparent contrast. To avoid this problem, the color in one entire bank should be the same. The easiest way to ensure uniform intensity and color is to replace all the bulbs at one time from the same case. Each case of bulbs will contain the same fluorescence characteristics. A bright light should not be used frequently or indiscriminately. An amperage meter (ammeter) should be installed so that light output is controlled and somewhat reproducible. High intensity may reveal some information in dark areas, but it overpowers information in less-dark areas.

Work Areas

Counters should be smooth, easy to clean, and cleaned daily. Hinged counters may be used as long as they are sturdy. Cabinets may be placed under and over the counters for storage. One drawer can be designated for holding repeat/reject films for counting at the end of each day.

File folder slots should be built in to remove the folders from the counter. Do not forget the convenient location of telephone and intercom. This area must be efficient and the work flow designed into the construction.

Smoking should be prohibited in work areas, since nicotine will stain the view-box glass and ashes can ruin films. The current interest in promoting clean air includes forbidding smoking in areas where nonsmokers work. Some hospitals have outlawed smoking entirely and refuse to sell smoking materials.

Work patterns should be organized so that film can be retrieved from the processor, be inserted into the file folder, and the folder returned to the correct compartment with the fewest steps. The film viewing area should be to the side of the film sorting area to reduce conflict of purposes and confusion.

Lighting

Lighting is very important since it affects the way we see and what we see. With a good view box and a radiograph, the eye receives a certain amount of information; but if there are bright ceiling lights, the eye will close down the pupil to control the amount of light. With a closed pupil, less light enters and a good film appears a little darker. It may give a false impression of an increase in contrast. The background lighting should be about 6 to 8 EV at ASA 100 on a light meter. Only view boxes covered with films (actual or black sheets) should be turned on, since the bright light will also affect the eyes. Bright light also causes more fatigue.

General Storage Requirements

Ambient Conditions

At all stages, x-ray film and chemicals must be stored under controlled conditions. The stages for film are receiving, bulk storage, darkroom storage, after exposure, and after processing. The chemical stages are concentrated and diluted. Film must be stored at 20°C (70°F) or cooler at all times to ensure the film will not be damaged. High heat deteriorates the film by exposing it and producing fog. The higher the heat, the sooner the film will become unacceptable. All films offer a 12-month expiration date, but this is based on the 20°C (70°F) level. Chemicals stored at higher temperatures will deteriorate more rapidly. Chemical concentrates will last about 12 months at 20°C (70°F), and the dilute developer about 2 weeks. At elevated temperatures, the life is greatly reduced. Dilute developer at 30°C (85°F) will last about 48 hours. Temperatures must be specified for all storage areas, verified at least monthly, and posted in a record book. Temperature tests include placing a thermometer in the chemical replenishment tanks at different times to be sure that they are not getting too warm. Thermometers and warning signs should be installed in the bulk storage area and long-term patient film storage. High temperature is a primary source of stain causing poor archival quality. Humidity for film must be controlled to a level of 40 to 60%. Below 40% relative humidity encourages static electricity buildup and discharge, marking the film; higher than 60% can lead to fog production. Relative humidity can be measured with a psychrometer (see p. 7). Film should be stored on the box edge to prevent pressure marks. All products should be stored using a first-in-first-out (FIFO) pattern: Film is placed on the right side of a shelf and removed from the left so that the oldest product is always used first. A complete documentation program is required so that product ordered from a dealer or from bulk storage can be accounted for. Finally, screens and cassettes must be stored on edge under the same conditions as film. Cassettes and unmounted new screens often are improperly stored or placed next to radiators, which can damage them.

Security

All green film should be kept under lock and key with careful inventory controls for two reasons. First, green film represents a sizable monetary investment. Second, film must be held in a secure environment to help protect it against conditions that could damage it. A damaged film will result in excess patient exposure, reduced return on investment, and reduced diagnostic quality. Documentation includes film brand, type, size, emulsion number, expiration date, and volume. Some institutions have found it advantageous to label or mark boxes of film with tapes or inks of various colors to help spot newer versus older product.

Inventory

Inventory involves a basic bookkeeping procedure that documents how much film is ordered, is received, and is in storage and in the darkroom. Film should be listed by brand, type, size, volume, emulsion number, and expiration date. As the film is used, meaning it is placed in the darkroom film bin, it is closed off the books. A second inventory program involves daily reconciliation of the amount of film left in a film bin (estimated), plus waste for the day (repeats and rejects), plus patient films. Monthly review should be made of the daily count versus invoices. Annual accounting is performed to determine if the volume of film purchased can be accounted for. At least a month's supply of film and chemistry should be within the institution at all times. New supplies should be automatically ordered to ensure that a month's supply is always in reserve.

Storage Areas

The receiving dock and area plus the bulk storage area are ideally under the direct control of radiology, but this is often impractical. Thus, radiology department personnel must educate and work with the purchasing, receiving, and stores personnel. Temperature, humidity, ventilation, stock rotation, stacking, and handling all must be reviewed initially and periodically. Isotopes cannot be shipped with or stored near film. Films and chemicals should not sit on a loading dock in the heat of a summer day or be stored near a furnace. Long-term storage of patient films is often relegated to the basement, where it can be hot and humid. The specifications call for storage of films at 20°C (70°F) and 40 to 60% relative humidity. As the seasons change and air-conditioners or heaters are turned on or off, the ambient conditions in all areas must be tested. An annual visit to dealer facilities to review stock and storage conditions is a minimal requirement.

Cassettes and Screens

Storage

Store cassettes on edge by speed of screen and size. Cassettes should be stored in slots or vertical boxes rather than laid flat. A stack of cassettes is precarious and may result in several sliding off onto the floor, becoming damaged. Cassettes are often stored in a pass box. The pass-box interior must be tested for radiation protection. Also, too many cassettes jammed into a pass box will result in their increased wear. An infrequently used cassette might remain in the pass box for many days. Cassettes should not be left loaded with film, because this can lead to artifacts and fog.

Labeling

Screens are provided with labels to be placed on the exterior of the cassette. These labels should carry the date of installation and should be covered with a clear plastic tape to protect them. The screen should be further identified with a permanent number placed directly on the screen so that it shows up on the radiograph. Although the screen contains a built-in serial number, this number plus the one added should be indicated on the cassette. Various cassettes containing different speed screens can be identified by colored tape or paint or by using code numbers. Records are required.

Cleaning

Screens must be cleaned weekly on a scheduled and documented basis. Screens, or more correctly the interior of the cassettes, should be brushed out or vacuumed out daily to remove lint and dust, which can cause white marks on the finished radiograph. The screens should be cleaned weekly with screen cleaner. If needed, antistatic solution may be applied. Never soak the screen with solution. Use a small but sufficient amount to cover the screen completely. Start at the top and work to the bottom, then go around the edges. Buff dry and stand the cassette up, and open it to further air dry for a few minutes. Next clean off the exterior of the cassette. Inspect the lead blocker area, edge felts, and hinges for signs of wear. Keep records on the total inventory, cleaning schedule, and any problems. Remove defective cassettes for repair.

Maintenance

Proper maintenance of cassettes requires that they be in a consistent state of good repair and usefulness. Thus, the first step is a thorough inspection each time the cassette is cleaned. If a cassette seems damaged or the lid seems warped or will not close properly during routine loading, then set it aside for inspection during a less busy time. Cassettes that begin showing signs of failure or fatigue should be repaired before they deteriorate to the point of being unrepairable or too expensive to salvage. Edge felts, hinges, and closure devices are usually the items to deteriorate first. Be observant of cassettes with blunted corners, which suggest they were dropped. Darkroom technicians and x-ray technologists have a daily responsibility to visually inspect cassettes as they work with them. A master file should be established and controlled by an assigned person. This responsible person is notified by cassette number of a potential or actual problem, and this is entered in the records. The cassette should be located and inspected. The maintenance records should help administration to plan for replacement purchases.

Inventory

Accurate records are required so that a defective cassette can be found, removed from service, tested, and repaired. Cassettes should be accounted for periodically, such as yearly or more frequently.

Testing

Testing should be made by visual inspection, mechanical operation, and radiographically. In this last case, use a wire mesh screen and cassette tester. It will indicate film-screen contact, sharpness, light leaks, dirt, and general screen response. The wire mesh is placed on top of a cassette loaded with film, placed on a tabletop. Try a variety of exposures to achieve a pleasing density level of about 1.00 to 1.50. Since viewing these wire mesh images is often fatiguing work in subdued background light, more than one person should review the films. Stand at least 0.61 m (2 ft) from the film—generally, the farther away the better. Another trick is to overlap two films and rotate them to detect patterns. Of course, one should always use one film emulsion, one exposure room, and the same processor for all of the tests. Record test conditions and results. Poor film-screen contact can sometimes be adjusted with a thin piece of screen foam.

Chapter 2

Chemistry of Film Manufacturing

Radiographic film is composed of a support base and emulsion layers (Fig. 2-1).

Base

Original photographic support bases were made of metal, but the earliest radiographs were on glass. It was optically clear and was devoid of casting streaks and bubbles, but it was fragile. Cellulose nitrate base in the early 1900s was about as good as the much thicker glass and was cheaper, but it easily caught on fire. Cellulose triacetate film offered a flexible, thin, clear support base that did not support or initiate combustion. However, it ripped like paper and under adverse storage conditions would dry out and shrink. Since the gelatin did not shrink, the film would pucker and cause a stained-glass effect. Present-day film support base is based on polyester technology developed by the Du Pont Company in the early 1960s. Polyester film base is a plastic that is optically clear, thin (0.107 cm [0.007 inches]), and stable to ambient conditions and processing conditions. In processing, the base does not retain moisture, aiding in faster processing time cycles. Polyester film base is found in most photographic applications today. The name *polyester* is a chemist's nickname or slang describing the fact that the product

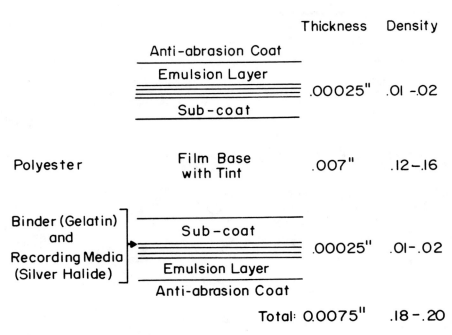

		Thickness	Density
	Anti-abrasion Coat		
	Emulsion Layer	.00025"	.01 -.02
	Sub-coat		
Polyester	Film Base with Tint	.007"	.12–.16
Binder (Gelatin) and Recording Media (Silver Halide)	Sub-coat		
	Emulsion Layer	.00025"	.01-.02
	Anti-abrasion Coat		
	Total: 0.0075"		.18 -.20

Fig. 2-1.   Cross section of radiographic film.

is actually polyethylene terephthalate ester. It is made by mixing dimethyl terephthalate and ethylene glycol, resulting in the growth of very long carbon chains that provide the pliability of the material, and thus it is a plastic. This reaction produces polyethylene terephthalate, and since the ethylene terephthalate has characteristics similar to a group of compounds called esters, its name becomes polyester. Du Pont introduced its polyester film base with the trademark name Cronar, and Kodak refers to theirs as Estar. The polyester is formed as a thick (0.64 cm [0.25 inches]) layer about 0.3 m (1.0 ft) wide; it then is biaxially (two directions) stretched until it is more than 102 cm (40 inches) wide and only 0.017 cm (0.007 inches) thick. When Du Pont innovated polyester film base, they also incorporated a blue tint in the film. This tint makes the blacks appear blacker and whites appear whiter, with an obvious apparent increase in contrast to aid in interpretation. The key word is *apparent,* since sensitometrically this is not true. The rather inefficient human eyes and mind are artificially aided by the tint. The tint also helps reduce eye fatigue, aiding diagnosis.

Emulsion

Once the film base is made ready to receive the emulsion by coating with an adhesive, the emulsion is coated on both sides of the base. The emulsion is composed of a binder and a recording medium consisting of silver halide crystals. The binder is composed of gelatin, which is manufactured from collagen. Collagen is a naturally occurring fibrous protein and is a major component of animal skin and bones. Collagen is treated with lime or an acid that breaks down the protein into a very pure gelatin. The gelatin has a great affinity for water—that is, it can absorb great quantities of water by swelling—and this is very important in the processing of film. To the gelatin is added a sensitized silver halide, which is usually silver bromide. Other useful members of the halide group are chlorine and iodine. The halide might also be combinations such as chlorobromide or iodobromide. The recording medium, silver bromide, is formed in this way:

(1) $2Ag°$ + $2NHO_3$ → $2AgNo_3$ + $H_2 \uparrow$
Silver + Nitric acid → Silver nitrate

(2) $AgNO_3$ + KBr → $AgBr \downarrow$ + KNO_3
Silver nitrate + Potassium bromide → Silver bromide + Potassium nitrate

The silver bromide is sensitized with a sulfur compound and mixed into the gelatin. Several washing operations follow until the emulsion is ready to be coated on the base. All of these steps must be carried out in total darkness. Once coated, the film base must be carefully dried, at which time the huge spools are taken to the finishing area. Here the spool is taken to the chopping operation, where the film is cut into specific lengths. These machines inspect the film and also count out the exact number of films for subsequent packaging in pouches and boxes.

Chapter 3

Sensitometry

Definition

Sensitometry is basically a metered or measured sensitization or exposure to a film. Of course, one cannot see the results of the exposure until after processing. Initially, this was a method by which, with controlled processing and a controlled (measured) exposure, a photographer could learn about the responses or characteristics of various films. Two British amateur photographers, Ferdinand Hurter and Vero Driffield, developed this system for characterizing the response of film to exposure and development. Their test procedure was important because it provided a systematic method for evaluating different types of films so one could take advantage of unique characteristics. What perhaps was not realized by Hurter and Driffield was the fact that for a given film and exposure, various processing chemicals and conditions can be evaluated or controlled. Also, for a given film and controlled processing conditions, various exposures can be evaluated. Thus, in summary, we find that sensitometry is a way to evaluate film, exposures, and processing. Sensitometry may be more precisely defined as the quantitative measure of the response of film to exposure and development. The key word for technologists is the word *and,* since the majority of their training is in exposure technique. Exposure, however, is only one factor or half of the system. Without development there is no image and, more importantly, improper development can alter the very best exposure. Indeed it can be further stated that development (or processing) controls image quality. If you use the very best film, screens, and exposure technique but development is inferior, an inferior visible image will be produced. It is very important that the average technologist be aware of this and that every institution have someone knowledgeable in processing chemistry and its control.

Hurter and Driffield found that by exposing the film to a range of exposures from very low to very high, with a uniform rate of increase, that the response in the form of density was not uniform. Thus they constructed a graph showing the stimulus (exposure) and the response (density). The curve that results is called a sensitometric curve, characteristic curve, or H&D curve in honor of the creators. By comparing curves of different film, one can better understand film differences and advantages. Sensitometry measures density (film blackening as a result of exposure and development), which has four values:

- Minimum density (D_{min}) for minimum exposure
- Maximum density (D_{max}) for maximum exposure
- Speed: a measure of the amount of exposure energy needed to produce a density of 1.00
- Contrast: a difference between two densities

Density

Definition

In a practical, everyday situation, density is defined as the amount of blackening or silver on the film. Indeed, as two radiographs are viewed for quality they have similar bases and tint, but if one is darker we say it has more density. This of course does not explain why it is darker. In a technical situation, we need to know the total density of film including the black metallic silver and the base density including tint. We measure density on a densitometer. This device passes light through the film and measures how much gets through. It then produces a value or density number. Density, mathematically, is the logarithm of the opacity or the inverse of the transmittance. Radiography is more concerned with the degree of transmittance than the degree of opacity. Transmittance, in turn, is the ratio of the intensity of the light incident (I_I) on a film and the intensity of the light transmitted or output of the film (I_t or I_o). The formula then would be as follows:

$$\text{Density} = \text{Logarithm } 1/T; \qquad T = I_0/I_I$$

$$= \text{Log } 1/I_0/I_I \qquad\qquad = \text{Log } I_I/I_0$$

The data obtained by sensitometric procedures are usually plotted in the form of graphs. Figure 3-1 is a typical characteristic curve of an x-ray film exposed with intensifying salt screens. The portion of the curve designated

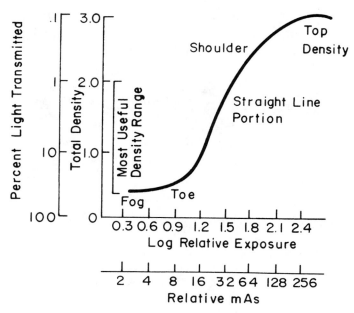

Fig. 3-1.   Sensitometric curve.

as the toe demonstrates the nonlinear response of the emulsion to relatively small amounts of radiant energy. With increases in exposure, the density builds up slowly until the linear response, or straight-line portion of the curve, is reached. Along this straight-line portion, the density increases uniformly with the logarithm of the exposure until the nonlinear shoulder of the curve is reached. The shoulder is not produced in industrial films with direct exposure. Additional exposure results in smaller increases in density to a point where additional exposure does not produce greater density.

Logarithms

When dealing with complex multiplication and division problems, it is often easier to use logarithms. The name is from two Greek words that mean symbols for doing arithmetic and is based on powers (exponents) of numbers. A logarithm can be generated based on any number raised to a power (multiplied by itself a number of times). The most common base number in nature (science) is 10, and these logarithms form the common "logs." In the equation $10^2 = 100$, we have multiplied 10×10 (read: 10 is multiplied by itself 2 times) to yield a product of 100. If we want to substitute a logarithm for the number 100, we would say: Based on a unit of 10 (common), how many times must it be multiplied by itself to yield 100? The answer is 2, which is called the characteristic. $\text{Log}_{10} 100 = 2$. However, many numbers are greater than or less than a whole multiple of 10, so we must use a table to give us a number to represent that portion. This is called the mantissa, and it is the same for every sequence of numbers arranged the same way. Consider the table below, which is based on common logs so the base unit is not written.

Whole Number		Characteristic	Mantissa (two to five places)		Complete Log
0	=	0	0	=	0
10	=	1	0	=	1.00
100	=	2	0	=	2.00
1000	=	3	0	=	3.00
3.192	=	0	5040	=	0.50
31.92	=	1	5040	=	1.50
319.2	=	2	5040	=	2.50
3192	=	3	5040	=	3.50

When one log is added to another, that is the equivalent of multiplying the whole numbers they represent; subtraction achieves division. In the above table, note that 319.2 is 10 times or one unit of 10 greater than 31.92. Since we are counting the units of 10, we say we have increased (31.92 to 319.2) by 10 times or 100% (one unit of 10 increase). Thus, the log increases respectively of 1.5040 to 2.5040 represent a 100% increase in value. It is important to understand this relationship when working with density, since density is a logarithm. There is seldom need to work with logarithms, but there is a real need to understand them. Returning to the definition of density:

$$\text{Density} = \text{Log} \frac{1}{I_0/I_1} \text{ or Log} \frac{I_1}{I_0}$$

We can construct the following table:

| Light Units | | | | Density | Log | |
I_1	I_0	I_0/I_1	Transmission %	I_1/I_0	I_1/I_0	Density
10	1	1/10	10	10/1	10	1.00
10	0.1	1/100	1	100/1	100	2.00
10	0.01	1/1000	0.1	1000/1	1000	3.00

The density scale represents the working range for medical radiography of 0 to 3.00. There is no unit value for density, so we write density (D) of 2.15 or D 2.15 or a density of 1.07 (D 1.07). Another common convention is to refer to density as optical density with the abbreviation OD, as in OD 1.07.

Measurement

Density is measured using a densitometer, which passes a known amount of light into the entire film and measures the amount of light emitting from the other side. It then filters the light with a yellow filter to compensate for the blue tint in the film base. This in effect nullifies the influence of the tint on the measurement. The amount of light is then converted to an electrical signal, which moves the pointer on an analog meter or displays the density number on a digital meter. Some analog meters such as the Mac Beth Quantalog series display density on the top scale and the percentage of transmission on the bottom scale. The densitometer must be calibrated every day it is used and zeroed prior to the reading of each film. Using the control strip provided by the manufacturer, the upper density level calibration must be verified or adjusted daily. The reading of 11 or 21 steps on a large exposure scale can produce sufficient data to construct a characteristic (H&D) curve. Another useful procedure is to select several exposure steps for spot checking of the density. Records and plus/minus charts are set up based on the limit of acceptability, which is the amount each density may deviate from a standard. Exposure systems can be produced by x-rays (or gamma) using an aluminum stepped wedge or by light flashed through a step tablet (sensitometer). In both cases, a gray scale is produced. The exposure system might have incremental exposure values increasing at a multiplier rate equal to the factor of 2 (2 times or 100%) or the square root of two ($\sqrt[2]{2}$), which is 1.41 times or a 41% increase. A third exposure found only on the Du Pont sensitometer uses the fifth root of two ($\sqrt[5]{2}$) exposure increment, which is 1.15 times or 15% incremental increase. Only a portion of this scale is used, and it is such a small increment and yet so sensitive that a person can make fairly accurate estimates of density variations just by viewing with the unaided eyes. The eyes cannot give density values but can determine approximate values and can certainly determine degrees of greater than or less than.

Values

As mentioned above, density has four values, sensitometrically:

- D_{min}
- D_{max}
- Speed: density level
- Contrast: difference of densities to enhance the visibility of details

It is often asked: What happens to the base plus fog (B + F) density value? and Isn't B + F a sensitometric value? B + F density is inherent in the film prior to exposure and, although it influences the visual quality and diagnostic clarity, it is not a part of the sensitometric values, which are based on measuring the response of the film to exposure and development.

D_{min}

D_{min} stands for the minimum density produced by the minimum exposure, and often the density value coincidentally equals B + F.

D_{max}

D_{max} is the density produced with the maximum exposure used but may not be the maximum density achievable by the film. Because of this, D_{max} is more correctly referred to as background density or top density or step 21 (on a 21-step exposure scale) density.

Speed

Speed is also referred to as the speed point but, more correctly, should be called sensitivity. Speed refers to the sensitivity of the film. A film that produces a density of 1.00 for a shorter exposure is said to be faster (this term originated with faster photographic camera shutter speed). A film requiring a higher exposure (longer time) is said to be slower and to have a lower speed. Films are referred to in terms of their sensitivity or speed—moderately fast, half speed, or high speed. The majority of x-ray film types used are in the moderate category. High-speed films are seldom used and therefore are relegated to special cases such as special procedures. Half-speed films are used with higher-speed screens to reduce noise characteristics. Half-speed films are growing in popularity. The density level of 1.00 is used because this represents a level where the eye is most sensitive. The word *speed* should only be used when discussing density values at the speed point level when comparing film. For instance, it is correct to say film A is faster since it has a speed point density of 1.09 (for a given exposure step) while film B is only D 0.98. On the other hand, it would be incorrect to say film A has greater speed in the shoulder, because speed is not measured in the shoulder of the H&D curve. Sensitometrically, speed is a density value. Speed may also be a value, a relative whole number that indicates the relative sensitivity of a film-screen combination. Medium-speed screens are assigned a relative speed value of 100. Using the same speed of film and a screen twice as fast would produce a 200 system, requiring half the exposure to achieve a density of 1.00 (speed point, approximately). Using the faster screen but half film would produce a 100 system again. System speed is based on the amount of exposure to produce a density of 1.00 on the film. System speed should not be confused with film speed.

Contrast

Contrast means difference. For two different exposures, two different densities are produced. Subtracting one density from the larger, second density produces a contrast number. The larger the number, the greater the contrast. On an H&D curve, the higher the number the steeper is the rise of the curve. The contrast number produced is the result of subtracting density values that are logarithms. However, the contrast number is not considered or treated as a logarithm but as a whole number.

D_{min} *Versus B + F*

D_{min}, minimum density for minimum exposure, is often referred to as B + F (base plus tint plus fog). B + F is inherent and not the result of exposure development. The base material has a density of 0.02 to 0.04, and tint has a density of approximately 0.08 to 0.10. Fog is the result of manufacturing processes and is a density of 0.01 to 0.02 per emulsion layer for a total of 0.04. Total B + F will range from OD 0.12 to OD 0.20 for a moderate-speed film. Of course, improper storage, age, heat, pressure, etc. all can result in an exposure that will be developed into noninformational density that is referred to as fog. Although fog is density, it is present prior to "normal" exposure and is not considered the result of the patient exposure. In general radiography, an indirect exposure system is used, meaning the use of salt intensifying screens. The film is not efficiently responsive to the lower levels of radiation or light, so the minimum exposure often does not expose the film sufficiently to show an increased density. Thus, coincidentally, D_{min} equals B + F in value although they are different measurements. In cineradiography and the newer modalities, camera systems are used and in general the rule is to make certain that D_{min} is measurable quantity above B + F to ensure sufficient exposure.

Indicated Versus Calculated

Indicated values include visual comparison ("eyeballing") of two films (a test film compared with a master) or spot densitometric readings (Fig. 3-2). In the latter case, several exposure steps are read on a densitometer and the density values are compared with those obtained by reading the same exposure steps on a master film. In either case, an indication of change or trends is provided, and that is often sufficient to alert the technologist to imminent problems. If a test film is similar to or matches the master film, then they are of equal value and control of quality has been documented.

Calculated sensitometric values, speed and contrast, must be derived from mathematical calculations using the H&D curve. Subtracting one density from another produces a difference (contrast), but this is only an indicated value despite the fact that a calculation was made. The reason is that the inherent B + F was not taken into consideration, and it affects different portions of the H&D curve differently. Thus, calculated values begin with the H&D curve and specific calculations are made, discounting the inherent fog (B + F) influence. Certainly calculated values are more accurate and provide

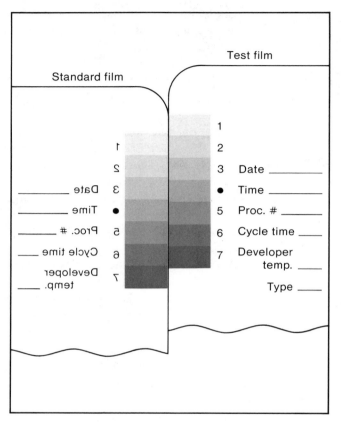

Fig. 3-2.   Visual comparison of speed point using $\sqrt[4]{2}$ visual step wedge.

better information than indicated values but are not necessary for a day-to-day effective quality control program. Calculated values become significant when communicating with other institutions or manufacturers since it provides a common language for understanding. Calculated values are performed essentially the same way by everyone. Indicated values will vary with individuals. Manufacturers' sales and technical literature always list calculated values.

Speed

Indicated speed is determined by selecting the exposure step on the gray scale that has a density close to 1.00. Calculated speed is determined by the amount of exposure required to produce a density of 1.00 net. ("Net" means after deducting B + F.) The Du Pont Company uses conventional H&D graph paper to which they have added a bit system scale that allows direct readings of calculated speed as bit values. Bit values are convertible into relative exposure (mAs) or arithmetic speed. Consult the *Bit System of Technic Conversion* for further details or Cahoon's *Formulating X-ray Techniques.*

Contrast

Contrast is indicated by selecting two densities and subtracting them. Quite often the low-density reading (D_1) chosen is the indicated speed point density. This is subtracted from a higher density (D_2) achieved with two steps higher exposure. The resulting mathematical difference is a contrast value. Another approach would be to select D_1 at two exposure steps below the speed point. The resulting difference in density is termed the delta D (ΔD) or contrast number. In the latter case, average gradient (a calculated value) is simulated; in the former case, gamma (a calculated value) is simulated. In neither case is the influence of B + F taken into consideration. Calculated values are based on the H&D curve with the following basic formula:

$$\text{Contrast} \ (\Delta D) = \frac{D_2 - D_1}{E_2 - E_1}$$

This reads as follows: Contrast (delta D or difference in density) is the density (D_1) produced by exposure number one (E_1) subtracted from the density (D_2) produced by exposure number two (E_2). In indicated values, specific steps (E_2, E_1) are selected; in calculated values, the density range or the exposure range may be selected or changed and is the net of the influence of B + F.

Contrast Calculations

Calculation may be made in several different ways to measure several different contrast areas of the H&D curve. These are gamma, gradient point, average gradient, and other units such as toe gradient, midgradient, and upper gradient.

Gamma

Gamma is a photographic catchword meaning contrast and should not be confused with the isotope radiation form. It is the measure of the steepness of the H&D curve along the straight-line portion (Fig. 3-3). It does not allow for toe or shoulder nonlinearity characteristics. Gamma is often used for industrial radiography, cineradiography, and general photography. To calculate gamma place a ruler along the longest, straightest part of the H&D curve in the center portion of the curve. Draw a line the length of the page. Move this line to the right and align the bottom edge to the contrast indicator built in the graph paper. Draw a new line parallel to the H&D slope line,

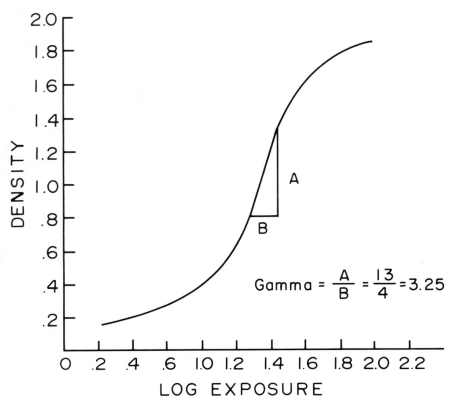

$$Gamma = \frac{A}{B} = \frac{13}{4} = 3.25$$

Fig. 3-3.   Calculating gamma.

and extend it until it cuts the vertical density scale. Read the value. This is the gamma (or contrast) value. Another calculation method is to determine trigonometrically the tangent of the angle of the slope line (drawn through the straight-line portion). The slope line is called the contrast line, gamma, gamma line, grade, gradient, or gradient line. Contrast is also called, based on the slope line, the slope or rate of inclination or the gradient. Measure the angle with a protractor, and look up the tangent of this angle in a table of trignometric functions. The number listed is the calculated contrast value.

Gradient Point

Gradient point is the opposite extreme of gamma (which measures the basic straight-line portion) in that it is the contrast measurement for any point on the entire H&D curve. The gradient point is selected for a certain density or a certain exposure level. For instance, a neuroradiologist might wish to know the contrast of the film (sensitometric/radiographic contrast) at a density of 0.90 for a contrast medium (radiopaque) fluid-filled blood vessel. Or, it might be useful to know how much increase or to what level contrast will change when a higher exposure is used. To determine the gradient point select the point and draw a line tangential to the point and proceed to calculate the slope (parallel lines or tangent of the angle) as described above (Fig. 3-4). It can be seen that there are infinite gradient points, so a contrast value must have its selection point stated, such as "film B has a gradient of 1.50 at OD 0.90."

Average Gradient

Average gradient is the average of all the gradient points that exist between the densities 0.25 and 2.00, which represent the range of usefulness. Since B + F must be subtracted, the coordinates for establishing the line become:

$$D_1 = OD\ 0.25 + B + F$$

$$D_2 = OD\ 2.00 + B + F$$

Adding in B + F causes the curve values to shift to the right, representing a subtractive effect. The curve does not move, but the resultant values are derived as if the curve were redrawn with B + F subtracted out. One method

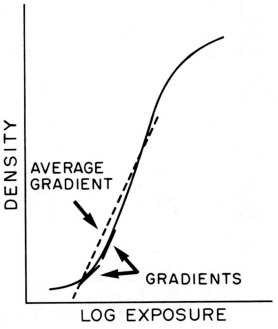

Fig. 3-4.   Average gradient or gradient points.

of calculation is the use the following basic formula:

$$\text{Contrast (average gradient)} = \frac{D_2 - D_1 = \Delta D}{E_2 - E_1 = \Delta E}$$

where D_2 is 2.00 + B + F and D_1 is 0.25 + B + F on the curve. This difference regardless of B + F value is always 1.75, which may be written ΔD 1.75. Where D_2 and D_1 intersect the H&D curve, read the log relative exposure value on the horizontal scale. Subtract E_1 from E_2 to generate a difference (ΔE). Divide ΔD (1.75) by the ΔE. The answer is the average gradient contrast value. Another method is to located D_1 and D_2 on the H&D curve and connect these coordinates with a straight line, creating an average slope line for all the gradient points (Fig. 3-5). Next calculate the value using the parallel rule method or tangent of the angle method discussed above under gamma. Another calculation procedure would be to create a right triangle using the slope line as the hypotenuse with D_1 and D_2 at the corners. Drop a vertical line from D_2, and label it Y; draw a horizontal line from D_1 to intersect with Y, and label it X. Be very careful to draw straight lines parallel to the graph paper lines and make careful subsequent measurements. Mea-

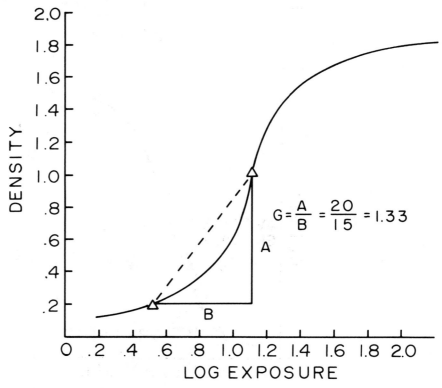

$$G = \frac{A}{B} = \frac{20}{15} = 1.33$$

Fig. 3-5.   Calculating average gradient.

sure in metric units. Divide the Y value by the X value to yield the average gradient value. A fifth method uses the bit scale built into the Du Pont H&D graph paper. In addition, there are nonograph overlays available. In all methods, the answers will be virtually identical. Average gradient is the most useful contrast measurement for general medical radiography. It is the value used in most technical literature.

Other Measures

Other measurements of contrast are toe gradient (the average between OD 0.25 and OD 1.00), middle gradient (the average between OD 1.00 and OD 2.00), and upper gradient (the average between OD 2.00 and OD 2.50). The measurements are not widely used but may grow in favor as technology makes better use of sensitometric values to produce the best diagnostic quality.

Practical Quality Control

The objective of quality control is to establish a system in which the quality of a product can be consistently maintained at acceptable levels. Both controls on controllable factors and tests of those controls are required. It has been said that quality control is only as good as the quality of the controls (tests). In a department with quality control, there is consistency, predictability, and confidence (Fig. 3-6). The components that go into a visible image are patient variations (subject contrast), technique selection (kVp, mAs, grid, film, screen, etc.), processing (time, temperature, chemicals, agitation, replenishment, etc.), and the viewing conditions (view box, background lighting, etc.). Of these factors, viewing conditions are the easiest to correct and control since frequent variation does not occur. Next would be processing, which has three basic factors: time, temperature, and activity. These may be monitored electromechanically (such as transport speed, temperature), chemically (such as pH), or sensitometrically. Of these tests, sensitometry offers the best tool since it represents the quality of the product being produced. All of the sensitometric values (D_{min}, D_{max}, speed, contrast) plus B + F, should be evaluated several times each day and recorded on a chart. Either indicated or calculated values may be used, but calculated are not required. The charts should include the date and time and should allow space for the tester's initials and any comments (Fig. 3-7). The object is maintenance of control; thus, it is necessary to establish parameters or limits of acceptability. These limits are usually plus and minus 15% for speed and plus and minus 10% for contrast. The midpoint is an arbitrary aim point. Data that over a period of time remain in the upper half or lower half or that swing vigorously up and down are not of concern if they are within acceptable

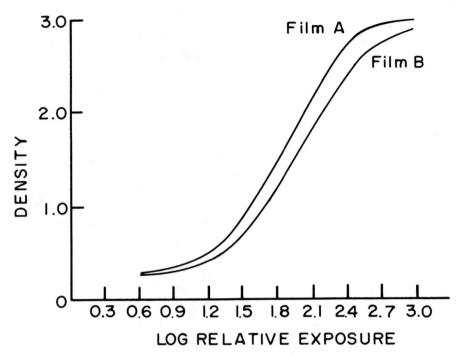

Fig. 3-6.   Comparing quality: speed and contrast shifts.

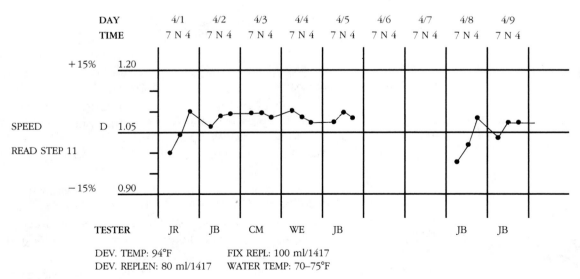

Fig. 3-7.   Trend chart.

limits. However, should the data begin to track obviously toward a limit or exceed a limit, then corrective action must be taken immediately. There should preferably be three tests a day: initially in the morning or at the beginning of a work shift, midshift, and at the end of shift or the end of the day at shutdown.

Tests consist of exposing a film from a control box of radiographic film set aside for testing purposes only. The exposure may be controlled by x-rays and screens using an aluminum stepped wedge or by use of a sensitometer. A sensitometer exposes the film with light through a step tablet of various shades of gray and is reproducible to a much greater extent than x-rays. The film is processed, reviewed, and recorded. No other action or tests are needed if the film is acceptable. If unacceptable quality is produced, then corrective action and retesting are required until the quality is again controlled. Record all observations, actions, and additional tests performed and the results (pH, temperature, clearing time, etc.). Always compare test films to the master film. Save all records on an annual basis. Review all data at least monthly. A more in-depth discussion of quality control trend chart construction and analysis is included at the end of this book.

Chapter 4

Processing

Processing Defined

Manual Processing

In the manual processing system, the film is placed on a hanger that is a metal frame of the appropriate size. In each corner there are spring-loaded pinchers consisting of a sharp point on one part and a hole in the second part. The point punches through the film corner to secure it. Two of these pinchers are spring loaded to put tension on the film to keep it flat. Hangers are loaded by beginning at the lower, fixed clip. Load one corner and move to the next fixed clip. Pull the film flat and clip it. Next slide the fingers along the frame, holding the film, to the upper spring-loaded clip. Pull the clip down and fasten it to the film. Finally move to the last spring clip and repeat. This pulls the film flat. The tanks for the chemicals are usually stainless steel and are placed inside a larger tank. The larger tank is filled with water at a desired temperature. This tank forms the rinse and wash tanks and provides the means of heating the chemicals. The chemicals usually are in sequence as follows: developer, rinse (short stop or acid bath), fixer, and wash (a final rinse). After the fixer, a hypo eliminator is sometimes used to aid washing. After the final rinse, a wetting agent is sometimes used to aid drying by helping the water to flow off the film. The technician places the loaded hanger in the developer, starts a clock, and agitates by raising and lowering the hanger rapidly. At the end of the development time, usually 3 to 5 minutes, the film is drained for 10 seconds or less (include this time in the development time) and is placed in fixer. If the first rinse or short stop is used, its functions are to stop development rapidly and to flush out developer and thereby prolong the life of the fixer. The technician fixes the film, washes it, and puts it into a dryer. In each step, the technician must fully submerge the hanger; provide vigorous agitation at the beginning, middle, and end of each time period; and carefully control the time factor. Time is most critical for development but becomes less critical for each subsequent step. A trained, efficient technician can process new films continuously or as fast as they can be loaded.

Automatic Processing

Automatic processing employs a machine termed a processor, which is an electromechanical (electrical and electricity-powered mechanical components like motors) device that provides transportation of the film, agitation, and temperature control. It even replaces consumed chemicals automatically. Inside the outer cabinet are found three tanks constituting the wet section (Fig. 4-1). They are sequentially the developer, fixer, and wash tanks. Next follows the built-in dryer. The time-temperature-activity factors are selected and set up in the processor by the processing specialist, quality control technologist, and/or the film manufacturer's technical representative. The darkroom technician simply places the film on a feed tray, aligning the film along one side. The film is drawn into the processor and is conveyed automatically through the unit until a dry film is deposited in the exit receiver bin. Roller

film path

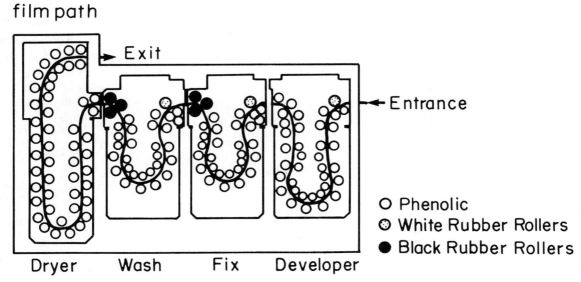

Dryer   Wash   Fix   Developer

O Phenolic
◎ White Rubber Rollers
● Black Rubber Rollers

Fig. 4-1.   Transport system.

squeegee action minimizes chemical carryover, and automatic chemical re-plenishment aids stability and uniformity.

Automatic versus Manual Processing

The automatic processing system offers only one real advantage over manual processing, and that is consistency. However, contrary to its name, it really is not automatic since it cannot measure sensitometric values and change itself (although the technology exists). The automatic processor is of limited automation and is as accurate as it is set up by a knowledgeable specialist. Automatic processing may be consistently good or consistently bad. Advantages such as personal safety, less mess, faster production, etc. do exist but are of no real value. Manual processing can be just as fast as automatic processing. Automatic processing developers contain a hardener to control film swelling. They also operate at much higher temperatures, which allow faster processing speeds and thereby higher capacities. It is fundamentally important to understand that processing is the conversion of the latent image into the useful visible image by a chemical reaction and is basically the same for all aspects of photography, especially black and white photography, which includes radiography. A processor is an electromechanical machine that controls various parameters of processing.

Cut Sheet Versus Cine

Cut-sheet processors are the most common. They accept a variety of film sizes from 10 cm (4 inches) long to 43 cm (17 inches) wide. They are not designed for continuous rolls or long strips, which have the tendency to tighten up rollers and overload the dryer. Cine, or motion picture, processors are classed as leader type, semileader type, or leaderless type. The exposed film is usually pulled through the chemicals by a leader. The film emulsion is usually positioned away from roller contact to minimize artifacts. However, the better cine processors use canted spindles or spindles with soft fingers that either do not touch the film image area or do so with very light pressure. Cut-sheet films are viewed directly; cine films are enlarged (blown up) on a viewing screen so that the smallest mark becomes objectionably large. The semileader system is a processor that uses a leader each time rather than always leaving the leader strung in the processor. In general, cut-sheet processor developers should never be used in a cine processor. After each use, assuming only one or two runs per day, cine developers should be drained out into a dark bottle, stoppered, and stored in a dark, cool place to help prolong the useful life. The electromechanical systems are the same in both units. One cine unit might process rolls 16 to 35 mm wide while another might only handle 35- and 70-mm rolls. Cine films are from 8 to 105 mm wide, so coordination between film size, camera requirements, and processor capabilities is required.

Function

Gurney-Mott Theory

Gurney and Mott developed their theory of how the latent image is formed, and, although much more is now known, their initial work described the foundation of latent image formation (Fig. 4-2). Understanding how images are formed helps one realize both the importance and function of the developer (processing). Beginning with the construction of a silver halide salt crystal, the crystalline lattice is composed of bonded silver and bromine. There is an excess of negative bromine ions (Br^-), which coat the outer surface, and an excess of positive silver ions (Ag^+) trapped inside, called interstitial silver. (Ag stands for silver and is an abbreviation of the chemical name *argent.*) The salt crystal is made more sensitive by adding a foreign compound called a sensitizer. At the moment of exposure, energy strikes the outer bromide ion (Br^-), and the excess electron in the conductance valence is split off, leaving bromine (Br^o) gas, which is absorbed by the gelatin. The liberated electron is trapped by the sensitivity speck, forming a sensitivity site, which is now negative. This causes interstitial silver (Ag^+) ions to migrate and pick up the electrons, becoming metallic silver (Ag^o). This is a self-

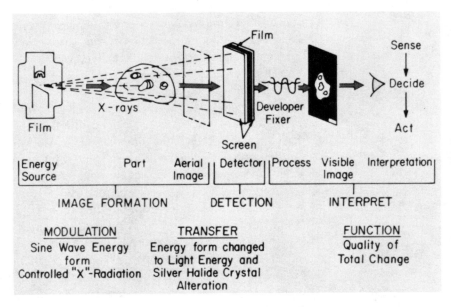

Fig. 4-2.   Radiographic systems.

completing reaction, once initiated by the exposure energy. If five atoms of silver collect at one site, a development site is formed. Without a development site, the crystal will not develop into silver. Thus the latent image is composed of exposed crystals containing minute piles of silver, at least five, and the equation can be written as follows:

$$AgBr + A^+ + \quad H \quad \rightarrow AgBr + Ag^0$$

$$\text{Unexposed} \quad \text{Exposure} \quad \text{Latent image}$$
$$\text{crystal}$$

This image is of no value until it is developed. The image is hidden. The developer makes the image—and all the technology it represents—useful.

Development of the Visible Image

The exposed film (crystals) is placed in the developer solution, which enters the gelatin. Halides in the film cause the developer to be oxidized, releasing electrons. These electrons enter the exposed crystals and attack the bonded silver bromide compound bonds. The crystals fall apart violently until all of the silver atoms are unbonded and formed into metallic silver. A developed single crystal that contained as few as five atoms of silver in the latent state now contains as many as one billion atoms. The amplication is approximately 10^9 times. The whole process is called an oxidation/reduction reaction. The developer is oxidized, and the silver halide crystal is reduced to basic metallic silver. This might be written as follows:

$$AgBr + Ag^0 + Developer \rightarrow Ag^0 + developer\ oxidized$$

$$\text{5 Atoms} \qquad\qquad\qquad 10^9\ \text{Atoms}$$
$$\text{Latent image} \qquad\qquad \text{Visible image}$$

If the developer or processing in general is not efficient, there is a direct relationship and effect on the final visible image. For this reason, it has been said that "processing completes what the exposure only started." Also, the developer has been consumed and needs to be regenerated and replenished. The developer efficiency is also influenced by time, temperature, and agitation factors, as are all chemical reactions. Development is stopped by the acid fixer, which in turn is flushed out by the wash water. The typical x-ray technologist has excellent training and daily involvement in latent image formation, and yet these are of little consequence if processing is not efficient, accurate, and optimal. It is not practical or even possible to produce diagnostic quality through attempts to overexpose and underdevelop or by underexposing and overdeveloping. Thus, processing must be understood and controlled.

Developer Consumption

Oxidation/Reduction Reactions

When a chemical is oxidized (broken down), it gives off electrons. The electrons are used to split another compound into a more simplified or reduced state—an oxidation/reduction reaction. A chemist might call it a redox reaction. The developer is oxidized; the silver bromide crystal is reduced to metallic silver. The developer contains reducing agents; the silver bromide contains the oxidizer. Something that is oxidized is often described as either broken down, depleted, exhausted, used up, killed, or burned up. Some examples would be rusting metal, a burning match, or a burned filament in an incandescent light bulb, fuse, or cathode ray tube.

Silver Development

During the development of the exposed crystals, containing development sites, the developer is consumed through oxidation. Specifically, the reducing agents hydroquinone and phenidone are broken down or changed into new compounds, and in this change there is a release of a multitude of electrons. The electrons attack exposed silver halide crystals, converting them to piles of elemental silver. The reducing agents have been destroyed and must be replaced so that the overall strength does not diminish, resulting in loss of film quality. It is understood that developer reducing agents are consumed at a rate based on the square centimeters (inches) of density. A larger film with a low average density level might consume equal or less developer than a smaller film with a high average density level. It is the function of the regeneration/replenishment system to replace the reducing agents consumed (activity regeneration) and to replace the solution carried out by the film (volume replenishment). If the replenishment rate is correct, the developer activity will not change and the tank will remain full—and this is the goal.

Aerial Oxidation

Oxidation or destruction of the developer reducing agents can occur by exposure to oxygen. Since this is not related to film silver development or regeneration, it is difficult to monitor and to correct. There are two common ways that aerial oxidation occurs: improper mixing and excessive standby operation. When mixing, the concentrated components (parts A, B, and C) must be added in proper sequence into water. Next, for each part, gentle mixing action is required. Violent or prolonged mixing will oxidize the reducing agents. Transferring developer by pumping or pouring should allow very little agitation and foaming. Replenisher chemicals must be stored in plastic tanks with both floating lids and dust covers. Floating lids keep fresh oxygen away from the developer. As the developer is pumped out of a replenishment tank, it acts like a giant piston, drawing in fresh oxygen. Instead of a floating lid, chemical minifloats or balls can be used in two layers. When oxygen in the air mixes with hydroquinone, the primary reducing agent, it causes an oxidation chain reaction, destroying the hydroquinone. Sodium sulfite is added as the preservative to stop the reaction through the formation of hydroquinone monosulfanate, which is a less efficient reducing agent. The object of mixing, then, must be to mix as gently as possible so that as little of the hydroquinone as possible is converted to the secondary product. Replenishment tanks must be placed where there is little chance of being bumped. Tanks should be placed away from heat and sunlight. Another common way in which the hydroquinone is broken down artificially is through prolonged heating and agitation within the processor in what is called standby. Many modern processors run normally but have a timer that will shut down various systems if a period of time passes and no films are fed into the unit. Standby mode may be manually or automatically activated. The processor might remain in standby mode until a film is fed or it might automatically cycle back to the run mode for a short period of time. In all cases, the developer solution is held at or near its usual operating temperature, and for this to occur there is usually agitation. Temperature and agitation will directly, measurably, and noticeably affect film quality through developer oxidation. Standby is a convenience device and not a quality control device. It is important to avoid allowing a processor to be in standby for more than 2 hours without developer replenishment.

Contamination

The developer will deteriorate if contaminated by other chemicals or heavy metals. The most common contaminator is fixer since it is close to the developer in the processor and can easily splash into it. For a 10,000-ml (2.5 gallon) developer tank, only 10 ml is required to deteriorate activity, and this amounts to 0.1%. Fume control hoods and splash guards must be used to help fight fixer fumes and splatter contamination. When adding fresh chemicals to the processor, always install the fixer first. If it splashes into the empty developer tank, simply rinse out the tank. Fixer contamination of the developer will result in the release of ammonia gas.

System cleaners based on sulfamic acid, dichromic acid, or sodium hyprochlorite (liquid laundry bleach) were originally designed to be used in long, narrow cine processor tanks, which otherwise are difficult to clean. However, those processors do not have rollers with hollow cores or with materials that would absorb or trap the cleaner. Systems cleaners may be used to clean the plumbing system but should not be used, or should be used carefully and infrequently to clean roller assemblies. If used on rollers, a weak solution should be poured over the rollers. Never soak the rollers.

System cleaners are hazardous and are not required. They function by hydrolyzing the gelatin that holds the dirt (silver) on the rollers. Water at about 40°C (100°F) works just as well.

Old developer such as that seen on the top of a floating lid in a replenishment tank or that left in the pump head of a processor after draining the system can deteriorate freshly prepared developer. Whenever it is suspected that developer is weak, it must be completely flushed out of all areas or it will weaken fresh, properly mixed developer.

Different types or brands of developers must not be added together. In some cases, there will be destruction of the fresh developer; in other cases, the foreign developer will alter the new developer to produce a third activity with unknown characteristics. Whenever developer brands or different types of the same brand are changed, make certain all tanks and lines are flushed and that the filters are cleaned or replaced.

Heavy metals such as copper or iron can adversely affect the developer by contaminating it. Non-stainless steel screws, paper clips, etc. might be used in an emergency to repair a processor rack, but keep in mind that these parts will corrode (oxidize) and can affect the developer. Seasonally, the metal content in public water supplies may change and can affect developer activity.

Development Control

Time/Temperature/Activity Relationship

All chemical reactions are controlled by one or all of these factors: time, temperature, and activity. Activity is a catch-all term that includes the general inherent activity of the chemical, agitation, moisture, and replenishment, among other factors. In manual processing, it is common to find literature discussing the time/temperature method of processing as superior to sight development. The implication is that the time/temperature method offers control whereas sight development is, by nature, variable—and this is a fact. Another aspect in manual processing is the realization that solutions are cooler than normal (20°C [70°F]) in the winter and warmer in the summer. The time/temperature relationship acts like a balance beam, in that when one is raised the other should be lowered to maintain balance. Thus, within a normal working range, if the temperature is too high or too low the development time is adjusted correspondingly, shorter or longer, to produce equal density. However, one important fact is often overlooked, and this is the activity of the developer. Different brands and types (from the same manufacturer) will have different activities and, therefore, different time/temperature values. The time/temperature balance might work less efficiently or not at all if the developer is weak or contaminated. Therefore, it might be summarized that in development there is a time/temperature relationship based on a given chemical activity. The time/temperature/activity relationship and the influence of these individual factors on speed and contrast are the basis for a manufacturer's processing guidelines.

Time Factor: Immersion in Solution

The only important time factor is the length of time a film is in the solution (developer, fixer, or wash). This is called the immersion time and is defined as the period of time from when the leading edge of the film enters the solution until the leading edge (same edge) exits the solution. In measuring this factor, use a smaller (8 × 10) film, which is easier to work with, but any size may be used. Make at least three tests. If rollers block the line of sight so the entrance and/or exit of solution cannot be seen, then this lost time must be deducted. One method is to measure the lost roller time on exit and/or entrance and mark the total distance back from the leading edge of the film (Fig. 4-3). Cut a small notch at this point, and feed the film into the rack assembly. When the notch enters the roller pinch point, start the stopwatch. The delayed action in starting the watch provides for deduction of the lost time. Stop the watch when the leading edge exits the rollers and is first visible. Another approach involves determination of the roller-to-roller time (gross time), measurement of the transport rate, measurement of time out of solution in rollers, and finally basic mathematics in which the lost time is subtracted from the gross time to yield net time. Modern processors include many with very short immersion times of 20 seconds or less. Should the calculation of the true immersion time be in error by only 2 seconds, this is a 10% error, which is visible on a film. Another problem is that developer

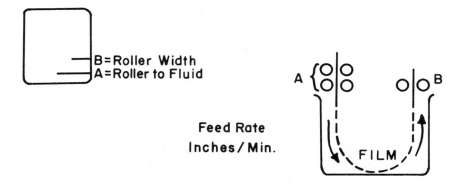

Example: Total roller to roller time = 23 sec.
Time lost in rollers out of solution 3″ at 1″/sec. = 3 sec.
Actual time = 23 sec. - 3 sec = 20 sec.

Fig. 4-3. Developer immersion time.

slowly leaking out through a valve or evaporating might result in a loss of only 1 inch of solution. The effect on the immersion time would be a loss of 1 second (based on typical 152.4 cm/minute [60 inches/minute]) on entrance and a loss of 1 second on exit, for a 10% loss. It can be a subtle variable. Immersion times should be known for each solution and recorded, as should solution levels. Solution levels should be checked at start-up each day and corrected if found to be low.

There are other factors that should be understood. Feed time is a factor of the overall transport rate (centimeters or inches/minute), the length of the film (feed time is measured as leading edge to trailing edge), and the time delay. Time delay in the activation of a signal (bell and/or light) provides a space so the next film will not overlap the first. Time delay is usually fixed at 3 seconds. It is an adjustable timer in some processors. The transport rate should be measured and recorded: Feed a 25.4-cm film into a roller. If it takes 10 seconds, then this translates into 2.54 cm/second (1 inch/second) or 152 cm/minute (60 inches/minute). Overall time can be measured as "dry to dry" or "dry to drop." The first is leading edge in (the feed end) until leading edge out (the last dryer roller). However, the film should not be touched until it drops free in the exit receiver bin, thus dry-to-drop measurement is both more accurate and practical. For this reason it is also called access time. Exit time will vary according to the length of film being measured, so this test should be standardized on one size.

Temperature Factor

All chemicals are basically temperature sensitive in that their rate of reaction increases as the temperature increases. This is true of developers, fixers, and the wash water. Higher temperatures mean that less time is needed. In addition to generally increasing activity, the higher temperatures swell the gelatin binder on the film so the chemicals can work more efficiently. However, too high a temperature will damage the gelatin, alter the sensitometric quality, and damage the chemicals. Temperature then is a very useful, easily manipulated, powerful tool that requires careful control and frequent monitoring. Temperatures are generally achieved by resistive heaters, and these are controlled by thermostats. To ensure uniformity of the solution temperature, agitation is required. Prolonged heating at a high 30 to 35°C (86 to 95°F) temperature with agitation contributes considerably to the oxidation and destruction of the developer and fixer. It causes water to evaporate and chemical fumes to deposit on rollers, making them dirty.

Activity Factor

Each brand and/or type of developer has an inherent activity level. If a certain time and temperature for development are chosen, such as 20 seconds at 30°C (95°F), one developer formula might produce a density level higher, lower, or the same as another brand or type. This general activity is not a measure of quality. Freshly mixed developer is generally too active (Du Pont's unique Cronex HSD high-stability developer is an exception) and will cause fog on the processed film. After dozens of films are processed, the activity will fall to a lower level that does not add additional fog. The lowering of the activity is due to bromide ions flushing out of the exposed film and collecting in the developer solution. The lowering activity is termed bromide depression. As the activity lowers, the temperature is raised to sustain a uniform density level. Because this was found to be so tedious, starter solution was invented. It is usually an acid solution (the exception is Du Pont's Cronex HSD, which uses a unique alkaline developer) containing bromide ions (pH 1 to 2.0, Br^- 4 to 10 gm/L), which simulates bromide depression. It is primarily only used at start-up when fresh chemicals are added to a new or cleaned processor. It is added at a rate of 20 to 25 ml/L (2.5 to 3.2 ounces/gallon). Brand A starter must be used for brand A developer and the correct quantities used. The manufacturer's processing recommendations are based on the assumption that this procedure has been taken. Thus starter solution is used to deactivate the fresh developer (it activates Du Pont's HSD developer) to simulate the eventual controlled state of activity.

Replenishment is necessary to sustain the developer at this controlled level of activity. For every square centimeter or inch of film containing density, there is a release of bromide ions and consumption of the reducing agents. To control the bromide ion accumulation (concentration) and its effect on overall developer activity and sensitometric quality, a fresh charge of replenisher developer is pumped in as a film is being developed. The replenishment chemicals have a higher pH and no bromide ions and therefore flush out or dilute the bromide ions. Correct bromide ion concentration is in a range of 4 to 8 g/L and is achieved with a replenishment rate of 80 to 50 ml/35 cm (14 inches), respectively. The higher replenishment rate will lower the bromide level, and the lower rate will raise the bromide level. The Du Pont Company Photo Products Department—X-Ray Technical Service (now called the Customer Technology Center for the Medical Department) developed a universal system for understanding and controlling exposure factors called the bit system of technique conversion. It is based on the photographic principles of exposure values. The Siemen's point system is similar. The bit (computer term for a piece of information) system assigns relative values (bits) to all components and factors that contribute to the final radiograph. A unique feature of the bit system is the ability to assign values to film-screen combinations, chemicals, and even processing. Optimal exposures are approximately 100 bits total. Optimal processing is 15 bits total. This is composed of time-factor bits plus temperature-factor bits plus activity bits. Activity bits are the relative activity of the developer brand and type. For instance, the Du Pont Company offers Cronex HSD with a bit value of 4.9. This is a high-contrast developer. Du Pont also offers Cronex moderate-contrast developer (MCD) with a bit value of 4.7 bits. This means that if a switch is made from HSD (4.9 bits) to MCD (4.7), the temperature would have to have raised to compensate for the 0.2 lower activity of the MCD (0.2 bits is the equivalent of a 15% exposure difference). In this way, films of identical density are produced but the contrast is different. The Du Pont Company has bit values for all chemical brands, and the system works regardless of brands or processors.

Agitation is important for efficient chemical reactions. First, the chemicals must be flushed through the gelatin to find all the crystals. Second, as development starts, bromides are released, as discussed previously, inhibiting further development. Agitation helps to flush away oxidation products and to ensure uniformity of development and of the developer activity because the replenisher chemicals are stronger and cooler. In a modern processor with a fast transport rate of 152 cm/minute (60 inches/minute), the rapid movement of the film is the primary source of agitation for complete development. The circulation pump provides agitation for uniformity of strength, temperature, and filtration.

Contrast Response Curves

For a manufacturer to determine guidelines for optimal processing, a series of tests must be performed. The manufacturer selects contrast as the most important sensitometric value to optimize. Next a series of films with controlled exposures are processed at different temperatures (30 to 35°C in 1°C increments [86 to 96°F in 2°F increments]). On a graph, the D_{min}, D_{max}, speed, and contrast are plotted according to temperature. As can be seen in the example below, there is an area where there is maximum contrast, and this becomes the point of optimal processing (15 bits). Any given institution might choose to operate on either side of the optimal point, and there are

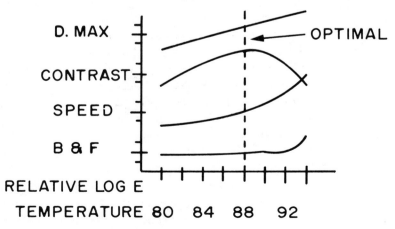

Fig. 4-4.   Contrast response curve.

valid reasons for doing so. Most institutions should seek out and operate close to the peak for contrast. This then is called a contrast (or gamma) response curve (Fig. 4-4). In photography, the word *gamma* is used to indicate contrast. This type of work is also called a gamma versus temperature curve. Similar curves may be produced by varying only time or by varying only activity. The curves produced all will be similar. However, in a hospital the only practical and easy test is temperature variation. This test should be performed by every institution. The slope of the contrast response curve will vary with different developer brands and types and with different processors. The shape might be hooked sharply and might be more critical or it might be a gentle curve and offer a broader working range. Although the manufacturer's recommendations are useful guidelines, it is very important for every institution to verify the data in its own processor.

Evolution of Time Cycles (History)

Since the advent of manual processing, which began in trays with the invention of photography, people have looked for a better way. In 1940–1955 came automatic hanger transport processors. These very large machines were automated manual processors. Film was loaded onto special hangers. The hangers were moved by conveyors to the developer tank and lowered in. A second conveyor moved the hanger through the solution. At the end of the tank, the hanger was lifted out and moved to the next tank. These processors worked on the same time/temperature/activity relationship as manual (3 to 5 min at 20°C [68°F]) and therefore required about 1 hour to produce a radiograph. In November, 1957, Kodak introduced a hangerless processor named the X-OMAT model M. It was advertised as a continuous roller transport assembly. Its most striking features were a much smaller size, absence of hangers, and faster processing. The original dry-to-drop time was about 15 minutes, or a fourfold increase in time. But the immersion time was still about 3 minutes. The time savings came from controlled time in the fixer, wash, and dryer chamber, which was much more efficient than manual drying cabinets. In the early 1960s, there was an explosion of processor makes. Most are no longer available or even in use. The X-OMAT became smaller, less complicated, and less expensive as it evolved. Pako, who used to make hanger transport units, introduced their Pakorol X model and then the slightly smaller XM model. Initially most processors had two developer tanks, but these were rapidly reduced to only one. Increased agitation and temperature permitted this. However, remember that film was not originally designed to be squeezed by several hundred rollers. Therefore, films and chemicals had to evolve to take advantage of the roller transport systems. Films were made with less gelatin and a harder surface; a hardener (glutaraldehyde) was added to the developer formula to control swelling.

In the early 1960s, the Kodak X-OMAT M4, Pakorol XM, Picker Pixamatic

I, Harper, Carr, and several others offered relatively compact units at reasonable prices. Hospitals, after cautious experimentation, gained confidence and found that these machines provided consistent quality. Time cycles were 7 minutes. This time factor for dry to drop is considered the standard. The developer immersion time was 2 minutes, and temperature was about 24°C (75°F).

In the mid-1960s, advances in film and chemical technology permitted these processors to double in speed, cutting the developer immersion time in half, to about 50 seconds. With the shorter time factor, temperature had to be increased to about 30°C (86°F). This was called the double-capacity cycle because the film capacity per hour was doubled with the doubled increase in the transport speed. The films and chemicals had to be changed to permit efficient operation under these conditions. This was called the 3½-minute cycle. It was introduced by the Du Pont Company, which did not market a processor at that time but converted any processor to the faster cycle.

In 1966, Kodak introduced the Rapid Processing (RP) system with the introduction of the X-OMAT M6. This unit was a speeded-up version of the M5, which was small in comparison to the larger-capacity and more expensive M4. The RP X-OMAT M6 (also referred to as M6-N or M6-NS) had 18 seconds of developer immersion time and operated at 40°C (103°F). However, temperatures above 40°C will adversely affect the chemicals and the gelatin. Films and chemicals were modified so that temperatures of 33 to 35°C (92 to 95°F) would produce sufficient density. RP is also called a fast-access (FA) system. Virtually all floor model and intermediate-size processors today are RP processing. This means they have 18 to 25 seconds of developer immersion time and require appropriate film and chemicals. The overall dry-to-dry time is about 90 seconds, so this is also called a 90-second cycle.

Many processors are found to take 98 seconds, or 120 seconds, or 105, or 110, etc. to produce a film. However, remember that the time cycle might be measured as dry to dry or dry to drop and will vary with film size. Also, overall time is of no practical consequence, since it is the developer immersion time that is significant. Thus, these slower 2-minute processors invariably will have developer immersion times of 20 to 25 seconds. This classifies them as 90-second class (RP processor class), requiring 90-second type film, chemicals, and appropriate temperature. The longer cycle time (access time) may be due to smaller overall size (tabletop units), which transports at a slower rate. It may be due to uniform (equal) rack length (and times), which increase the margin against error in the fixer and wash (less fixing and washing time are required than development time). It may be due to a longer dryer chamber. A typical large floor model 90-second processor with staggered racks might transport at a rate of 152 cm/minute (60 inches/minute), while a tabletop processor that is smaller and may have uniform rack length may transport at only 50 cm/minute (20 inches/minute). Remember that the important factor in image quality is developer immersion time, and not the feed rate, access time, transport rate, or general processing class. All cycles are based on the immersion time in the developer because the temperature and film and chemistry must match.

Processing Versus Processor

Definition

Processing is accomplished by means of chemical reactions (development, fixation, washing) that produce the useful visible image. Processing, like all chemical reactions, is controlled by time, temperature, and activity factors and relationships. A processor is an electromechanical collection of support systems that control time (transport system), temperature, and activity (replenishment system, circulation system). Thus the processor exists for the sake of the chemistry. There are six processor systems. In processing, there are seven systems, which include the six processor systems plus the chemistry system (developer, fixer, and wash). Another point of clarification is that the correct terminology is *processing monitoring* rather than *processor monitoring,* since the latter is subordinate to the former. It is processing quality control that is vital to optimal diagnostic quality. Indeed, sensitometric quality control is to measure how processing affects a controlled exposure on a controlled piece of film.

Processor Systems

1. The transport system controls the time factor. It is composed of two subsystems: the conveyor and the drive. The conveyor subsystem handles the film and moves it along with rollers and deflector plates. The drive subsystem includes motor, gears, sprockets, and chain. It is the energy to move the rollers.
2. The temperature control system is also called the tempering system. It controls the temperature of the developer, fixer, wash, and dryer. It is composed of heaters controlled by thermostats. Sometimes it includes passive heaters/coolers called heat exchangers.
3. The circulation/filtration system circulates the chemicals for uniform activity and temperature plus filtration to remove debris. It is composed of pumps and tubing.
4. The replenishment/regeneration system replenishes volume and regenerates the activity. Film sensors activate a pump to inject fresh chemicals from a storage tank.
5. The dryer system removes moisture from the film so that it can be handled. The system includes one or more blowers, heaters, thermostats, and an exhaust duct.

6. The electrical system is obviously a part of all the other systems, but it can be discussed alone as a separate entity.

These six systems are found in all photographic processors. Understanding them in one type of processor allows the technologist or service person to be able to work with any photographic or radiographic processor.

Processing Systems

Since processing is a chemical reaction controlled by time/temperature/activity relationships, the seven systems are the six electromechanical systems of the processor plus the chemical system. The chemical system includes the developer, fixer, and wash. The developer activity is stopped by the fixer. The fixer, in turn, must be washed out to prevent damage. The functions of the chemicals are as follows:

Developer: Swell the emulsion layers.
             Reduce exposed silver bromide crystals to black metallic silver.
Fixer: Stop development (neutralize the developer).
             Clear away all remaining silver halide crystals.
             Shrink and harden the emulsion.
Wash: Swell the emulsion.
             Dilute out all chemicals.

Ambient Conditions of the Processor

The chemical tanks are often stainless steel, which convects heat easily. These tanks are inside the processor. When the processor is closed up with its decorative side panels, cover, and shields, it becomes very hot inside. The internal ambient conditions are very hot (40°C [104°F]) and humid (80% relative humidity). The ambient conditions surrounding the processor may be only slightly different from the rest of the institution. Thus when working on the processor or troubleshooting, keep in mind that the inside conditions are much more harsh than those found on the exterior in the light room. Modern processors use plastic tanks to provide better insulation against the internal ambient heat. Modern films generally dry at much lower temperatures, so the ambient temperatures are lower also.

Chapter 5

Chemistry System

The number system that indicates the relative acidity or basic nature of a chemical is known as the pH scale. The symbol *pH* means the exponential (p) value of hydrogen or hydroxyl ions available for a reaction. Those chemicals having a high hydrogen potential (H^+) are called acids. Those having a high alkaline potential (OH^-) are called bases. If unity or 1.0 represents the strongest acid, then a weaker acid would have to be a value less than 1.0. This could be 0.1 and the next could be 0.01, and these values can be expressed using powers (exponents): $10^1 = 1$, $10^{-1} = 0.1$, $10^{-2} = 0.01$, and so on. At 10^{-14} we have reached the weakest acid. Writing 10^{-14} as a whole number would involve many zeros to the right of the decimal point. Simply using the 14 indicates the weakest acid and the strongest base. At this level, it is the strongest basic chemical, which, based on alkalinity, would be a pH of 1.0. The two scales cross at pH 7.0, which is the midpoint of both scales. Thus, one scale may be used instead of two. The pH scale ranges from 0 to 7 (acids) and 7 to 14 (bases). It is very important to remember that the pH scale is logarithmic based on powers of 10. A pH of 4 is 10 times or 100% stronger than a pH of 5.0, and a pH of 5.0 is half as strong as a pH of 4. The pH scale development might be as follows:

Hydrogen ions available: pH scale for H^+

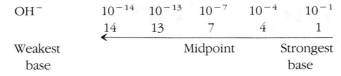

Hydroxyl ions available: pH scale for OH^{-1}

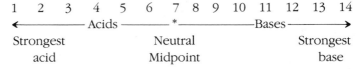

Combined scale

| 1 | 2 | 3 | 4 | 5 | 6 | 7 | 8 | 9 | 10 | 11 | 12 | 13 | 14 |

←————————— Acids ————————— *————————————Bases————————→

Strongest   Neutral   Strongest
   acid   Midpoint   base

The pH scale indicates the relative acidity or alkalinity of a chemical. It is also important to realize that the difference between one level of pH and the next is a power of 10, 10 times, or 100%. Thus, when mixing concentrated components together it can be appreciated why the proper sequence must be followed. The pH is only a relative indicator of processing chemical quality. Sometimes the pH will be correct but the result will be unacceptable and vice versa. Measurement of pH is best performed using a temperature-compensating pH meter. The meter must be buffered (zeroed) to the approximate level to be read. For instance, zero the meter to pH 10.0 using a known buffer solution when measuring developers. Buffer to pH 4.0 when measuring fixers. The reason for temperature compensation is that the higher the solution temperature, the higher the pH. The pH should be measured with the temperature at 20°C (70°F). Most pH papers are of little value. The more expensive color-corrected, narrow-range papers are generally accurate but are accurate only to plus or minus 15%.

Specific Gravity

Specific gravity measures the relative weight or density of a solution when compared with water at 23°C (72°F). Measurement is made using a hydrometer and a hydrometer stand or graduate. The specific gravity or density of water is 1.000. Developers fall in a range of 1.070 to 1.100, whereas fixers range 1.077 to 1.110. When mixing developers, a quantity of water is added to the mixing tank, which is often the replenisher tank. These tanks change shape and become distorted. As the tank distorts, the volume of water added may be in error. Making a simple hydrometer test will indicate if the correct water dilution has been made. For instance, if a correctly diluted developer has a density of 1.070 but the hydrometer reads 1.063, this indicates about 10% overdilution. Overdilution will weaken the chemicals. Underdilution can be corrected by adding additional water. Usually, manufacturer's specifications allow a margin of ±0.004. Remember to control the temperature to 23°C. Also, when purchasing a hydrometer be careful to buy one with the narrowest range rather than a broader range. The hydrometer stand is shaped like a graduate (long cylinder) with a larger top, which acts like a reservoir. The hydrometer is placed into the stand filled with chemicals. Never drop the hydrometer into the stand. The hydrometer will float. Sight across the meniscus (surface) of the solution to read the specific gravity. Used developer will average 1.080 to 1.100, or about 1.090, as a result of evaporation of water.

Development

Developer Function

The function of the developer is to convert the latent image into the visible image. In so doing, the developer is consumed (oxidized) and the exposed silver halide crystals are reduced to metalic silver. The development action results in amplification of the exposure signal by as much as 10^9 times. The development action is controlled by time, temperature, and activity factors.

Developer Components and General Functions

Reducing agents reduce the exposed crystals to metallic silver. Hydroquinone is the primary agent. It works slowly to produce the blacks of the shoulder of the H&D curve. Phenidone works rapidly, producing the gray tones.

The reducing agents are activated by an alkaline medium such as sodium carbonate. The alkaline medium also helps to swell the gelatin in the emulsion layer to help ensure that the developer gets to all crystals.

To control the activity of the reducing agents, an antifoggant is added. The antifoggant reduces the activity of the reducing agents to protect unexposed crystals from being chemically attacked and subsequently converted to silver. If unexposed crystals are chemically exposed, the resulting density is termed chemical or development fog. Fog is the single most common and deleterious artifact in radiography. Fog is noninformational density that covers the entire film. The chemical name for the function of the antifoggant is *restrainer*. The traditional antifoggant is potassium bromide (KBr), which is an inorganic compound. Modern formulas use organic antifoggants such as

6-nitroimidazole or phenylmercaptotetrazole. Better-quality developers contain as many as three different restrainers.

Water is the solvent. Drinking quality is the only necessary standard for the water used. Water hardness, parts per million (ppm) of dissolved minerals (carbonates), should be in the moderate range (40 to 150 ppm), which includes most drinking water supplies.

To help control the swelling of the gelatin in the emulsion, a hardener is added to automatic, cut-sheet processor developers. Controlling the amount of emulsion swelling aids in transportability and the amount of chemicals taken up by the gelatin. If overswelling occurs, the result is inefficient fixing, washing, drying, and transport. Glutaraldehyde is the general developer hardener used.

Reducing Agents

In modern radiographic developers, there are two reducing agents: hydroquinone and phenidone. Although hydroquinone has always been used, phenidone was used only when processing advanced to shorter immersion times and corresponding higher temperatures. The original combination was hydroquinone and metal (or elon) and was called an MQ developer. Modern chemicals are referred to as PQ developers. Hydroquinone is abbreviated HQ or Q. Another name for hydroquinone is quinol. It is a benzene ring with two hydroxyl groups.

Phenidone works very fast and develops (reduces) those crystals found in the lighter exposure areas. If a series of exposed films were processed at 5-second intervals with temperature and activity held constant, the graph in Figure 5-1 could be plotted. Notice that the phenidone plateaus and ceases

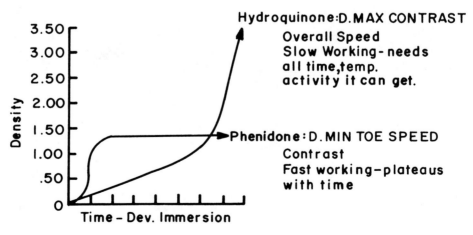

Fig. 5-1.   The effect of reducing agents on sensitometry.

producing density although higher densities exist. Phenidone controls the grays of the H&D curve and thus is the influencing factor over the toe region of the curve. Sensitometrically, phenidone controls the minimum density (D_{min}) and is the primary controller of speed (film sensitivity).

Hydroquinone works more slowly in reducing those crystals in the heavier exposure areas, the black areas. Processing exposed films in an alkaline solution containing just hydroquinone, with a changing time factor, would produce a general nonresponse at first, followed by a sudden shoot upward. This can be seen in Figure 5-1. Note that since the hydroquinone affects the blacks primarily, it controls the shoulder of the H&D curve and sensitometrically controls the D_{max} and is the primary controller of contrast. The hydroquinone is easily oxidized, so it is the weaker of the two reducing agents. Thus, D_{max} and contrast are usually the first variables to show indication of developer failure (see Fig. 5-1).

In processing exposed films in the proper combination of hydroquinone and phenidone, it would seem logical to get a combination of effects or an average effect based on the graph shown in Figure 5-1. But a unique phenomenon occurs in that the two together produce a result that is not predicted by simply adding together or averaging the independent effects. Furthermore, the effect is greater. This is called a synergistic effect, which is defined as the whole being greater than the sum of the parts. In chemistry, the word used to describe this condition is *superadditivity*. In medical radiography, we would find little use with H&D curves shaped like those produced by phenidone or by hydroquinone. That is, we cannot use high speed with no contrast (phenidone) or high contrast but very slow speed (hydroquinone). The superadditive result is a low D_{min}, high D_{max}, average or better speed, and high contrast. This, of course, is the best possible combination (Fig. 5-2).

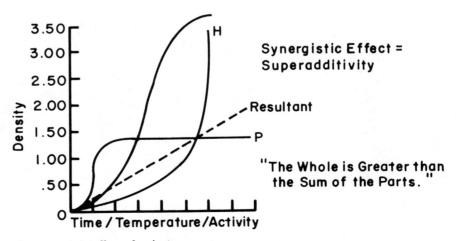

Fig. 5-2.   The synergistic effect of reducing agents.

The hydroquinone is easily broken down by heat and air, such as in prolonged periods of standby; by excessive heat in mixing, storage, or in use; by mixing that is too violent or prolonged; and by being contaminated with fixer, old developer, or heavy metals. Of course, normally, the hydroquinone is consumed as it is oxidized to produce electrons, which are used to produce the visible image. The amount of hydroquinone (and developer in general) used in the silver development work is based on the square centimeters (inches) of density. A large film with a low exposure (which results in a low density) will consume a certain volume of developer. A smaller film with a high exposure producing high densities might consume an equal or greater quantity of developer. When a film is entered into a processor (this is termed *feeding*), it activates a film detection mechanism that turns on a pump to inject fresh developer to replace that which is consumed by the redox reaction and carryout. Replenishment maintains the volume and regenerates the activity. When oxidation or contamination occurs, it is unrelated to film size or density so the developer is weakened. No compensation is made. The first movement of the sensitometry will be a lowering of the shoulder and then a side movement to the left, with a rise in toe fog.

It is very difficult and expensive to analyze hydroquinone, and thus it is often done without charge by the manufacturer of the film or the chemicals. Hydroquinone determination is in grams per liter (g/L). Fresh developer contains 20 to 30 g/L depending on brand and mixing efficiency. Used developer contains 15 to 25 g/L. Abused developer contains 10 to 12 g/L. In the clinical situation, the best tool is sensitometry. By monitoring contrast and D_{max}, it is possible to detect failure early. Frequent tests are required. Normally, phenidone need not be tested or worried about.

Activator

Activator usually is an alkaline medium such as sodium or potassium carbonate or hydroxide. pH levels of 10 to 11 are common, with working solutions in the processor closer to pH 10.0 and from 10.0 to 11.0 in manual processing. Usually (except for Du Pont Cronex HSD) the replenisher pH is about 0.3 higher. The pH is not an indicator of developer strength or quality. Many things affect the pH, such as bromide ion buildup and temperature.

The activator provides a medium necessary for the reducing agents to work. Also, the alkalinity swells the gelatin binder in the emulsion to help ease the reducing agents in finding all exposed crystals.

The activator might be depleted by bromide accumulation from films and underreplenishment. Bromide levels should be 4 to 8 g/L. The activator is carried out from the film into the fixer. This is controlled by the roller squeegees and the developer hardener. Common ways to deplete the activator are to weaken it by overdilution with water, contamination with acid fixer or systems cleaners, or underreplenishment. Monitoring with a pH meter might be useful, but only in trying to solve a problem. Daily testing is not required.

Antifoggant

The standard antifogging agent is KBr, which is preferentially attacked by reducing agents instead of the unexposed crystals. If the unexposed crystals were attacked, they would be chemically exposed and developed into silver. This silver would not be a part of the information, so it is noninformational density or fog. Thus there is a need for an antifoggant, which a chemist would call a restrainer. Modern antifoggants/restrainers include 5-methylbenzotrazole, 6-nitrobenzimidazole, benzitriazole, and 1-phenyl-5-mercaptotetrazole.

Antifoggants are adsorbed to unexposed crystals to protect them from the reducing agents and thereby are consumed. Aerial oxidation also affects them. Overdilution with water in mixing or underreplenishment weakens them. The best tool is sensitometry, which shows a left-moving speed shift as the antifoggants deplete.

Preservative

Sodium sulfite is the preservative of choice. Its function is to preserve the hydroquinone by controlling aerial oxidation. Hydroquinone in the presence of oxygen begins a chain reaction in which hydrogen is robbed and the hydroquinone is oxidized into semiquinone and quinone. Each one of these steps is indicated by the formation of brilliant blue and red, respectively, so that totally oxidized developer often appears green, or like used motor oil. Sodium sulfite stops the chain reaction of destruction by linking with the oxygen and hydroquinone to form a new compound called hydroquinone monosulfanate (HQMS). Once the oxygen is consumed and HQMS has been formed, further oxidation ceases. To help ensure that fresh oxygen is kept away, floating lids are required in the replenishment tanks, excess agitation must be avoided, and heat should never exceed 23°C (75°F) in the replenishment/storage tank.

In mixing fresh developer, hydroquinone levels of 30 g/L in the concentrate will be reduced to 25 to 27 g/L, with the production of an equivalent 5 to 3 g/L of HQMS. Excessive or violent mixing, mixing in the wrong sequence, or excessive heat might result in an unacceptable HQMS level of 10 to 15 g/L.

If the preservative is depleted, the hydroquinone will become oxidized, resulting in a loss of the H&D shoulder with a loss of D_{max} and contrast. Sensitometric testing is the best tool, however some manufacturers will perform chemical analysis of developers to determine the integrity of the sulfite.

Solvent

Water is the solvent, and it usually must only be of drinking quality. No specially treated water is required. It should be filtered to at least 40 micrometers (μm, microns) for cold-water use and to 5 to 10 μm for tempered-water use when a mixing valve is employed. The lower level is to prevent jamming the mixing valve. The limit the unaided eye can see is 40 μm. Dissolved solids should be less than 250 ppm, pH should be 6.5 to 8.5, hardness should be moderate (40 to 150 ppm), heavy metals (copper, iron, etc.) should be less than 0.1 ppm, chloride less than 25 ppm, and sulfate less than 200 ppm. Most tap water supplies in North America fall into these ranges. Well water will vary depending on whether it comes from a shallow or deep well and the amount and types of chemicals needed to treat it to meet health requirements. Abnormal water supply will directly affect the chemical activity. Most manufacturers of film and chemicals and water treatment companies can perform analysis. All city water departments perform routine testing and have quality control personnel who can give advice. These experts may not know how a particular water situation affects radiographic developer, but they usually know how black and white (B&W) photographic developers will be affected. Radiographic developers are specialized B&W developers.

Hardener

To control swelling of the gelatin in the warm alkaline developer and to allow passage through the various rollers and turns, a hardener is added to cut-sheet automatic processor developers. The hardener used is glutaraldehyde, which is of the aldehyde family like formaldehyde (which is often used to harden films in manufacturing). These chemicals are often thought of as tanning agents because they cross-link long protein fibers to make a tight weave, with the result that animal skin is turned into more durable leather. The gelatin of the emulsion is protein, and it is cross-linked to prevent excessive swelling.

The hardener is packaged in an acid medium, which it favors. Upon mixing, it is blended into the high-alkaline medium of the developer solution and begins to deteriorate. It is very difficult to test glutaraldehyde concentration, so testing is by observation and inference. If the hardener becomes marginal or depleted, any or all of the following problems can occur: plus density (wet pressure sensitization, scratches, pressure lines, fog, scuff marks), minus density (scratches, pick-off, scuff marks), uncleared film (milky green), failure to transport (jams) or maltransport (slipping, cocking), poorly washed films (high hypo retention), and wet films. Developer hardener failure is primarily the cause of unclear films and/or wet films. The fixer hardeners are seldom at fault. To determine which chemical is at fault, perform a clearing time test (see the fixer section). If the clearing time is adequate, then the fixer is adequate and the developer, by inference, is at fault.

Brand Characteristics

Each brand (manufacturer), and even different types of developers from the same manufacturer, must be characterized as to their general activity level. For instance, the time/temperature relationships are based on a given chemical activity. If the immersion time is 20 seconds in the developer at 33°C (90°F) for brand X but brand Y requires 35°C (95°F) to produce the same density (speed), it is concluded that brand Y has a lower inherent activity. It cannot be concluded that brand Y is of lesser quality, because that is not true or indicated.

Each institution should perform an evaluation to determine the developer brand characteristics using the temperature versus gamma response curves. Sensitometrically exposed films (all the same exposure and same emulsion) are processed at 2° temperature intervals from 30 to 36°C (85 to 96°F). On a graph, the D_{min} or base plus fog (B + F), D_{max}, speed, and contrast values are plotted versus temperature. From this chart, the operator can calculate optimal contrast/speed ranges and determine the developer's response characteristics. Of course, the technologist can always seek the recommendations of the manufacturer. However, keep in mind when seeking this advice to ask for the recommendations based on the types and brands of film used, brand and model of processors used, developer immersion time, and brand and type of developer used.

The Du Pont Company, as a part of its bit system of technique conversion, has tested and assigned relative activity values to most types and brands of developers. Contact the local representative.

Developer is a very inexpensive part of the cost factors needed to produce a diagnostic radiograph. The best developers should be used, and consideration should be given to using film and developer from the same manufacturer.

Mixing Procedure

The vast majority of developers are liquid, but there is some interest in returning to powders to control shipping costs. Liquid "put-ups" started out as powders and crystals that were blended in a chemical plant, which is set up and staffed differently from a radiology department or office.

Liquid put-ups usually contain three parts. Sometimes part A is found in two bottles or two parts. The basic parts specifications to make 76 L (20 gallons) of solution:

Mixing Sequence	Part	Component	pH	Quantity	
				Liters	Gallons
1	—	Water	6.5–8.5	53	14.0
2	A	Hydroquinone Preservative Activator	11–12.0	18.9	5.0
3	B	Phenidone Antifoggant	3.0	1.9	0.5
4	C	Glutaraldehyde (hardener)	3.0	1.9	0.5
			10–11	75.7	20.0

Begin and end each mixing operation with clean equipment for personal safety and to prevent contamination. Rinse and wash mixing paddles, tanks, lids, funnels, etc. each time before use, even if they look clean, and as soon as the mixing is complete. Ideally, separate paddles and tanks should be used for developer and fixer. Be observant to keep lint, hair, and pieces of the cardboard boxes out of the mixing tanks. All oxidized developer must be wiped off tank walls and washed from floating lids and dustcovers. The outside of the tanks should be kept clean, since unclean surfaces attract and hold dirt.

Cylindrical tanks can be calibrated mathematically, but this does not take into consideration the distortion of the tanks as they are filled with chemicals that weigh about 3.6 kg (8 pounds) per 3.8 L (1 gallon). When a 114-L (30-gallon) tank is filled, there is about 109 kg (240 pounds) of pressure on the tank walls, which will distort. As the tank is being filled, the tank walls bow, causing a change in the diameter and thus in the capacity. The preferred procedure is to calibrate the tank using a calibrated vessel such as a bucket from a laboratory supply company. As known quantities of water are added to the tank, mark the volume on the outside. Marks molded in or stenciled onto new tanks cannot be relied on. Calibration should be performed quarterly. Square or rectangular tanks distort less.

Tanks can be of any size or shape to fit into work areas. Tall, narrow tanks (round, square, rectangular) save floor space, reduce surface area exposed for aerial oxidation, and help control head pressure variation on the replenishment pumps, but it may be difficult to fit them under a counter. Low, wide tanks would easily fit under a counter but may be harder to work with. The best solution is to know that there are many alternatives, and the work area should be carefully planned.

Mixed developer should be bottled and capped to prevent aerial oxidation, or, if it is in a replenishment tank, a floating lid or two layers of minifloats (balls) should be used. As the developer is used, it acts like a giant piston drawing in fresh air, which contains oxygen. A floating lid keeps the oxygen away from the developer and helps preserve the hydroquinone reducing agent.

Dustcovers keep dust, lint, hair, and waste materials out of the tanks. Such debris probably would not affect the developer, but it will clog filters and damage pumps or alter the pumping rate. Dustcovers must be loose fitting. If they were airtight, no chemicals could be pumped because a vacuum would develop.

Mixing sequence, noted above in the components list, is extremely important because of the pH of the concentrates. Alkaline part A must be diluted in water before the acid parts B and C are added. It is trite to say, but the rule is always to read and follow the directions that are on or with the chemical concentrate package. The primary reason is to ensure that the person mixing chemicals does not start taking shortcuts or doing it their own way. Another reason is that the manufacturers might make a small formula change calling for 1 or 2 L more water (0.5 gallon).

In chemistry, the one rule for mixing solutions is always to start with the lightest component and add subsequent heavier solutions. Water should be placed in the tank first, followed in sequence by concentrated parts A, B, and C, with intermediate mixing. These concentrates are much heavier and will fall through and blend into the water. Pouring water on top of concentrates is like pouring water on a hard surface. As the water splatters, it carries some concentrate, which can cause chemical burns. Thus for purposes of safety and chemical integrity there is a saying: Always add *A*cids, *B*ases, and *C*oncentrates into water. Radiographic developers also contain parts A, B, C, which should be added to water in sequence.

Agitation is important to blend the various chemicals. Excessive, violent, or prolonged mixing is to be avoided since this leads to oxidation and a loss of quality. Blending part A into water will be evidenced by an oily appearance. When fully blended, the solution will be clear. Never use a garden hose at full blast to inject water or use the force of the water for mixing. This action results in greater oxidation and hazards.

Storage and Inventory

Concentrated and/or dealer-prepared "ready-mix" (premixed) must be inventoried to ensure adequate supply and stock rotation for freshness.

Some chemical manufacturers stamp concentrate boxes with the date of manufacture. Others use a code that indicates the month and year of manufacture. These codes can be useful to help ensure that the oldest chemicals are used first. In addition, a simple code using the month, day, and year can be added by the institution to control inventory. Ready-mix brought to the institution by the dealer and placed in storage should be dated by the institution's representative. Personnel charged with obtaining and emptying these containers into replenishment tanks should be instructed to use the older material first.

Inventory control is economically justifiable. It helps indicate whether or not solutions are being wasted and if what is purchased relates to what is consumed.

Concentrated chemicals should last about 12 months when stored at 21°C (70°F). The higher the temperature, the shorter the life. At 40°C (104°F), the concentrate might last only 1 month. Cooler temperatures are preferred and have no effect, down to 5°C (40°F). Very cold environment may result in crystallization or precipitation. This problem is usually corrected on warming up to room temperature.

Diluted developers, correctly prepared, should last about 14 to 21 days in the replenishment tank. If no fresh developer is added within that time, then discard the remainder. Flush the tank, the replenisher and circulation lines, and processor and refill with fresh. If fresh developer is added, then the activity will be sustained. Storage should be at 15 to 21°C (60 to 70°F), with a floating lid and dustcover. Agitation, bumping, and sunlight are to be avoided. Periodically, especially at the end of the day, check the temperature in the replenishment tank. At 30°C (86°F) the developer will last about 7 days; at 35°C (95°F) the developer will last about 48 hours. Overdiluted or improperly prepared developer is weaker and will fail more easily.

Safety

The developer is a very hazardous chemical solution, primarily because it is usually considered to be not dangerous since it is alkaline. The pH that is the most destructive to the eyes is pH 11.5, with a broader range of pH 11.0 to 12.0. Concentrated part A is pH 12.0; dilute developer is pH 10.0 to 11.0. Hydroquinone can be absorbed through the skin, so avoid regular or prolonged contact. Hydroquinone as a powder or dust is very corrosive to the membranes of the eyes and nose. Glutaraldehyde is a tanning agent. The United States Occupational Safety and Health Administration (OSHA) advises that the handling, mixing, storage, transport, or use of hazardous chemicals requires policies, teaching programs, and safety equipment. Only trained personnel should perform mixing, cleaning, or maintenance work, and they must use eye protection. An eyewash station should be prominently displayed wherever developer is mixed, stored, or used. This includes such areas as outpatient, surgery, shipping and receiving, and storerooms, as well as in radiology. In addition, rubber gloves and an apron should be worn.

Should developer get into the eyes, wash them with running water within 15 seconds and continue washing for 1 hour while a doctor is called. Do not stop washing, and do not administer any medications.

Radiographic chemicals are not available to the general public. They are sold only to professionals for a specific purpose. Unfortunately, there may be people using these products under the loose or nonexistent direction of a professional. Thus the opportunity exists for an accident. In 1986, new regulations established by OSHA, the Environmental Protection Agency (EPA), and the Department of Transportation resulted in dramatically improved and expanded labels under the "right to know" legislation. These new labels include a list of hazards and first aid instructions. In addition, OSHA material safety data sheets (MSDS) that contain other technical data are available from the manufacturer. The user is required to have MSDS sheets on hand for all chemicals used by employees. As of October 17, 1987, the EPA SARA-Title III requires all users of developers to report the quantity.

Solution Service Chemistry

A solution service company prepares several hundred gallons of a product at one time, reducing the cost. In many instances, processor maintenance, repair, and silver recovery service all are tied together in a package. The chemicals generally are correctly prepared, but because of their influence on an institution's exposure technology, it is the responsibility of the institution to challenge and test this product periodically via quality control. Sometimes problems go undetected or uncorrected by the dealer and are not detected until many films are repeated in the institution. The problem is that the institution made an assumption of integrity without testing to prove integrity. Many dealers do their own testing and sampling. Indeed, when a problem occurs, it is usually institution related rather than dealer related.

The institution's processing specialist, quality control technologist, administrator, and/or other interested persons should develop a series of checks and balances including testing of dealer-prepared developer. These persons should annually visit the dealer facilities and discuss mutual objectives and procedures. This effort is directed to preventing problems. Incidentally, when solution service personnel work within a contract institution, they should follow that institution's safety practices or policies unless their own are more restrictive.

All chemicals should be in color-coded and labeled containers. As containers are received, they should be inventoried and dated.

Starter Solution

Components

Starter solution is primarily acetic acid at a pH of about 2.0. The major exception is the starter for Du Pont's HSD, which is alkaline. Starter also contains bromides, usually in the form of KBr.

Function

Starter solution is used when fresh developer is added to a clean processor; it is used at start-up, and thus the name. Its function is to simulate the eventual steady state or "seasoned" condition of the developer. As exposed films are processed in developer without starter, the film releases bromides as the exposed crystals are reduced to metallic silver (Fig. 5-3). There generally are no bromides at first, but they build up slowly to a level of 4 to 8 g/L. At this level they act as a restrainer and lower the effect of the reducing agents. Normal or seasoned developer contains 4 to 8 g/L of bromides. The problem is that from fresh to seasoned represents unacceptable change, and the higher activity of fresh developer results in chemical fog.

Types and Quantity

Starter is added at a rate of 19.5 to 25 ml/L (2.5 to 3.2 ounces/gallon) to fresh developer to deactivate it (or to activate, in the case of Du Pont's HSD), to simulate its eventual condition and preclude change. Starter can be added into the developer tank at any time. It is very important always to use the same brand of starter as the brand of developer. Different starters have different bromide levels.

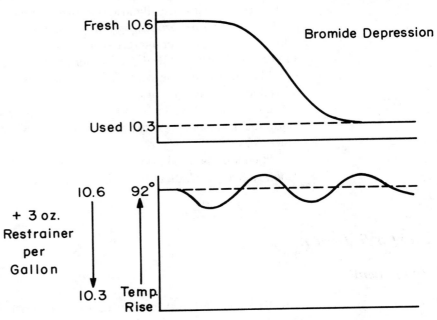

Fig. 5-3.   Starter solution purpose.

Short Stop

Function

Short stops are only used in manual processing. They serve to stop developer action rapidly, to help control fog and stain production, and to prolong the life of the fixer. Of these functions, prolonging the life of the fixer is the most important. If the bulk of developer is diluted out of the film prior to fixation, the fixer life will be prolonged.

Components and Types

Short stop bath may be water, a weak solution of fixer, or an acetic acid bath. It might be a prepared solution or simply formulated by the user.

Fixer

Fixer Function

The clearing or fixing agent is ammonium thiosulfate. The former agent was sodium thiosulfate, which was also called the hyposulfite of soda, from which came the nickname *hypo*. Thus, the term *hypo* is used to indicate the entire fixing solution (tank, rack, process, etc.) and, erroneously, ammonium thiosulfate. The activator is acetic acid.

Preserving the chemical equilibrium is accomplished by using sodium sulfite, the same preservative found in the developer.

The hardener is usually an aluminum compound such as aluminum chloride or potassium alum.

Clearing Agents

Sodium thiosulfate is no longer in use as hypo because of the shorter times and higher temperatures of modern automatic processing. However, it functioned basically the same as its successor, ammonium thiosulfate.

The primary ingredient is the clearing agent, which is also called the fixing agent, or ammonium thiosulfate. Its function is to dissolve the silver out of the remaining silver halide crystals, both exposed and unexposed. By clearing away these crystals, the mechanism for capturing an exposure is removed so the film is fixed against further exposure. The ammonium thiosulfate picks up the silver to form a new compound called ammonium thiosilver-sulfate complex.

The developer forms deposits of silver that make up the visible image, and the fixer washes out all remaining cream-colored crystals so that the less-dense areas appear white in comparison. Radiographs are most usually read as a transparency. Without removing unexposed crystals, it would be more difficult to see the information contained in the density. The thiosulfate clearing agent also helps in stopping the developer action.

If the fixer is weak, the developer is not rapidly stopped and some overdevelopment fogging occurs. This will appear as toe fog but is actually uniform over the entire film, constituting a speed shift to the left (increase). In addition, if the film is not completely cleared, it becomes more difficult to read the film. Also, inefficient fixing can lead to dichroic or hypo retention stain, and either one renders the film questionable or useless.

The fixer is primarily depleted by inadequate replenishment to combat carryout and dilution due to developer carry-in. Silver accumulates in the silver thiosulfate complexes, diminishing the ability of the thiosulfate to clear more silver out of the film. These complexes are broken down and the thiosulfate regenerated by the preservative, sodium sulfite. The sulfite is weakened by overdilution, underreplenishment, and the use of recirculating electrolytic silver recovery units. Measurement by chemical analysis of the thiosulfate level is not practical. An inference to its efficiency can be made by performing a clearing time test (Fig. 5-4). Most 90-second type films should clear completely in good fixer in less than 10 seconds at room temperature (as in the replenishment tank) and in less than 7 seconds at 30°C (89°F).

FIXER TIME FACTOR

Fixer Time = 2 x Clearing Time

Example I : "90 Sec." Type Film
"90 Sec." Type Fixer
Clearing Time = 7 Sec
x 2

Fixing Time Total I 4 Sec

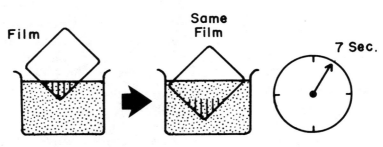

Fig. 5-4.   Clearing time test.

The clearing time test is performed in white light with a piece of typical green radiographic film (preferably fresh from a film bin). A strip about 5 cm (2 inches) wide and 10 cm (4 inches) long can be used or the corner of 20- × 25-cm (8 × 10 inches) film can be used. Dip a portion of the film into the fixer until a clear patch is seen. Next, submerge this part and more of the dry green part into the solution. Gently agitate until the second patch is as clear as the first patch. This is timed with a stopwatch. When the second patch matches the first patch, no additional time is necessary because the two areas match and the first patch had extra time to clear. Perform three tests and calculate the average to eliminate the effect of error. This test is perhaps the single best indicative test for chemistry. It is simple and indicates if the fixer is working. If the clearing time is adequate, it may be assumed that all other factors are also adequate.

Activator

The activator is acetic acid. The pH is between 4.0 and 4.5 for a used, steady state (seasoned). The activator's functions are to provide an acid medium for the hardener and to neutralize the developer.

As alkaline developer is carried into the fixer via the film, the activator is somewhat neutralized and the pH moves from 4.0 toward 4.5. Also, as silver is dissolved in the fixing action, the pH is altered. Normally adequate replenishment will sustain the pH at 4.5. If the activator is weak, then some overdevelopment fogging will occur.

The pH level can be measured using narrow-range pH paper or a temperature-compensating pH meter buffered to 4.0.

Preservative

Sodium sulfite is used to preserve the fixing solution by keeping the thiosulfate in equilibrium. This is the same preservative used in the developer. The sodium sulfite dissolves the silver out of the silver thiosulfite complexes and regenerates the thiosulfate so it can clear away more silver.

If the silver thiosulfate complexes are not dissolved because of weak preservative, the result is increased chance of hypo retention stain production and an unclear film. The sodium sulfite can be depleted by excess developer carry-in, which dilutes the fixer, underreplenishment of the fixer, and/or the use of recirculating electrolytic silver recovery units. Recirculating units plate out the silver through electrolysis (passing electrical current through a solution), but this also destroys the sulfite preservative. Thus, with the use of recirculating recovery units, lowering the replenishment rate below 80 ml/35 cm (14 inches) should be avoided. Improper mixing will also affect the preservative.

The preservative can be measured in grams per liter and should be in a range of 15 to 50 g/L.

Hardener

Aluminum compounds such as aluminum chloride work very well on protein chains, which make up the gelatin binder of the emulsion. The aluminum chloride drives out the moisture, shrinks the emulsion layer, and hardens the surface. Another hardener is potassium alum.

The hardeners are generally packaged in strong acids (pH 0.5 to 1.0) to keep them in a nonviolent state. If they are blended in too rapidly, the concentrate causes a reaction that will precipitate sulfur and aluminum. Careful and slow blending of the hardener is important. Vigorous agitation should be used. There is no way to determine hardener efficiency other than by inference using the clearing time test. When a processor produces wet films, the fixer is usually suspect; however, more often it is the developer hardener that has failed. When the developer fails to control swelling, the overswollen film cannot be compensated for by the fixer hardener. On some occasions, such as replenishment pump failure, both the developer and fixer will be weakened so that both contribute to wet films or jams.

Time/Temperature/Activity Relationship

The immersion time is twice the clearing time. If the clearing time is 7 seconds, then a minimum of 14 seconds is needed for complete fixing. This means that in the first half of the time the film is cleared; in the second half, the swollen film is shrunk and hardened. The gelatin of the emulsion layer is very ionic sensitive. The gelatin loaded with developer enters the acid fixer and actually swells dramatically and rapidly. The fixer hardener must shrink the film as a result of the developer swelling and the gelatin fixer swelling. Most processors provide approximately 10 to 30% margin for error in the total fixing time.

Temperature increase from 20 to 30°C (70 to 86°F) will increase the rate of clearing. The temperature should never exceed the developer temperature, and temperatures from 35 to 45°C (95 to 113°F) will result in overswelling of the emulsion beyond the capability of the hardener to control. Fixer temperature should be monitored at the end of a day or whenever wet films are a problem. Processors with stainless steel tanks for the fixer can easily accumulate excess heat.

Activity is expressed as agitation, which improves the clearing rate about 10% but is of limited value. The pH should be between 4.0 for fresh fixer or replenisher and 4.5 for stable, used fixer. Sulfite, as noted above, is consumed by electrolytic recirculating silver recovery units, by overdilution (by water during mixing or by developer because of underreplenishment), and by improper mixing (adding part B too rapidly).

Safety

Properly diluted fixer is not particularly hazardous in pH or toxicity. Part B, containing the hardeners, at a pH of 0.5 to 1.0, is an extremely strong acid that is considered corrosive to skin. Always wear protective equipment on the eyes and hands. Should contact occur, wash vigorously with copious amounts of water. Follow the mixing instructions exactly.

				Quantity	
Sequence	Part	Component	pH	Liters	Gallons
1	—	Water	6.5–8.5	53	14.0
2	A	Ammonium thiosulfate Sodium sulfite Acetic acid	5.0	18.9	5.0
3	B	Aluminum chloride Acetic acid	$\frac{0.5}{4.1}$	$\frac{3.8}{75.7}$	$\frac{1.0}{20.0}$

Specific gravity: 1.070–1.110

Always start and end with clean equipment. Wash tanks and mixing paddles prior to use, even if they look clean. Place the required amount of water at the correct temperature (20°C [70°F]) into the mixing tank. Pour in part A and blend until clear as water. Slowly add part B. If adding is too rapid, yellow stain will be seen where the chemical hits the mix. Pouring slowly against and around the inside of the tank often helps distribute the chemicals. Mixing may and should be very vigorous but should not cause splashing. Follow the instructions with the concentrate. Periodically, just prior to mixing a fresh batch, stir up the bottom of the tank to see if there is any precipitation, which is aluminum. If found, discard the solution and flush the tank clean. Precipitation is the result of adding part B too rapidly and/or high storage temperatures.

Add fresh fixer to the clean processor first. If any fixer splashes into the developer tank, it can be easily flushed out. Splash guards can be fashioned from discarded x-ray films.

Storage

See the above section on developer storage. Avoid heat, rotate stock, and keep an inventory.

Hypo Eliminator

Function

In manual processing and in some automatic cine processors, a hypo eliminator is used directly after the fixer. Its function is to flush out the hypo (thiosulfate complexes) to make washing easier and sometimes faster. Another benefit is insurance against hypo retention or archival stain. Hypo left in the film can damage the film in storage by producing yellow/brown stain, which is silver sulfide (Ag_2S).

The usual formula is a mild acid solution containing sodium sulfite, which is the fixer preservative and a solvent of silver. By ensuring that much of the silver thiosulfate complexes are broken down to silver and thiosulfate, there is more complete washing and less chance of stain production. Hypo eliminator is not needed in automatic cut-sheet processors because of squeegee rollers and the developer hardener, which control gelatin swelling and the amount of chemicals absorbed.

Washing

Chemical Function of Water

As mentioned above, the fixer's thiosulfate must be washed out of the film to prevent stain. The Ag_2S stain is formed by a reaction of silver and thiosulfate. Leaving silver thiosulfate complexes in the film only makes the chemical reaction easier. Washing out the thiosulfate is easier than washing out silver. Thus, the water must wash out most of the thiosulfate. Should Ag_2S stain form in the film, it will be a pale yellow stain at first that, when combined with the blue base tint of the film, will appear green. As the stain intensifies it becomes more yellow, then amber, and finally brown.

A film is retained in long-term storage for the patient and for reference by the medical staff. The period of time is usually 5 years but will vary from 3 to 40 years after death. Archival quality requires that documents remain unchanged (or at equal quality) for a period of time. The American National Standards Institute (ANSI) suggests in their standard for hypo retention (pH 1.41–1976) that the level not exceed 8 $\mu g/cm^2$ (25 $\mu g/inch^2$). Usually, a modern film processed in adequately fresh chemicals will easily meet this goal. However, in cold-water processors the cold water is less efficient so the amount of retained thiosulfate will be larger. Warmer water washes more easily and effectively because of the gelatin swelling action. Agitation is very important and that is why a large volume of water 4 to 11 L (1 to 3 gallons) is used. Newer processors (e.g., Du Pont's QC1 R/T) use a water circulation pump to conserve water and yet provide sufficient agitation. If the developer and hardener become weakened, especially the developer hardener, this will affect the archival quality even with normal and sufficient washing. The diminishment of the fixer preservative, sodium sulfite, also results in poorer archival quality.

Quality

Water should be of drinking quality. This is important because it is used in great quantities. The rate per minute is not great, but on an hourly, daily, and monthly basis it becomes a large quantity. Water solenoids and optimizing washing can greatly reduce consumption. However, the lack of need for special water (i.e., distilled, etc.) is an important economic consideration. Also, slightly dirty water actually increases washing efficiency. Hardness should be moderate, at 40 to 150 ppm; pH should be between 6.5 and 8.5, although it will drop a little as fixer is carried into it. Dissolved solids should be less than 250 ppm. The specific gravity of water at 23°C (75°F) is 1.000.

Time Factor

Time is fixed at 50 to 100% of the developer time. If washing is inefficient, then temperature should be increased since time is fixed. The wash immersion time should be determined as a base figure for future reference.

Temperature Factor

Temperature has a direct effect on gelatin swelling, and this directly affects washing efficiency. The water temperature usually should be as warm as possible but never greater than 3.8°C (5°F) less than the developer temperature unless so directed by the processor manufacturer. The reason is that water has a mechanical function, discussed below.

Agitation

Agitation is very important and is accomplished by passing the film through the solution and by the water flow rate, which may be supplemented with a pump for greater agitation. Spray bars (e.g., Assisorio Radiographico of Milan, Italy, EK M-8) also work well but are seldom used.

Mechanical Function of Water

Water is used to help control the developer temperature. In a few processors, the water is the source of developer heat. In the majority of processors, however, the water must be 3°C (5°F) less than the developer temperature so that it "steals" heat. By removing heat, the thermostat and heater cycle on and off more rapidly. All solutions (and gases, such as air) that are heated electrically suffer from overshoot and undershoot. An uncontrolled heater becomes more efficient with a thermostat, but there are inherent inefficiencies that permit the temperature to drift to 1 to 2°C (2 to 3°F) over and under the desired set point. To combat this, cool water is placed in close proximity to the warmer developer with a steel wall between them. This device is called a heat exchanger. Heat is convected to the cooler side, the thermostat responds more rapidly, and overshoot and undershoot are reduced to an acceptable level of ± ¼ to ½°C or F. Thus, the wash water has a mechanical function to control the developer temperature.

Balancing Chemical versus Mechanical Function

The larger the difference (Δ) in temperature (T) (delta T = ΔT) between the water and developer, the lower should be the volume. A 20°ΔT might need only 4 L/minute (1 gallon/minute), whereas a 5°ΔT might need 12 L/minute (3 gallons/minute) to effect the same exchange. The colder the water, the better the mechanical function but the less effective is the chemical function of washing the film for archival quality.

The first step in making any changes in the water supply characteristics is to request a hypo retention analysis from one of the film manufacturers. Based on the analysis, intelligent decisions can be made to balance the two water functions.

Combating Algae and Bio-Slime

Algae are found at most times in the air and in the water as microscopic spores. These spores are like seeds, in that when conditions are correct the spore begins to grow into a "flower." The algae grow and attach themselves to the tank walls, rollers, fittings, and drain lines.

Bio-slime is a slimy mass that feels similar to algae and is the result of bacteria cells finding a proper growth environment and growing simple one-cell creatures that build up layers. The living layer kills off the underlying layer, causing the slimy feeling. Bacteria are present at most times in the air and in water.

The traditional method of preventing algae and bacteria from growing and coating tank walls and/or rollers was to run the water continuously, breaking up the fragile growth before it became a heavy layer and flushing it away. This approach did not work all the time and overlooked the cause of the problem, in addition to being expensive. Water at 3 gallons/minute does not seem like a lot until it is considered on an annual basis. Three gallons per minute is 180 gallons/hour, 1800 gallons in a 10-hour day, and more than 50,000 gallons/month. If the water is heated at all, the cost escalates.

Today there is a need to conserve resources and energy and to eliminate waste in business.

Algae and bacteria grow because they have an environment consisting of the right moisture, food, and warmth. These are found in the wash tank. Food is in the form of protein in the gelatin and thiosulfate carried into the wash tank by the film. Whenever the water stops flowing, such as at the end of the day, the water becomes stagnant and growth can begin. Because the water tank is the source of heat in manual processing and is near the warm dryer in an automatic processor, the water is generally warm. Another phenomenon occurs in automatic processors that have stainless steel tanks: When the processor is shut down, the interior ambient heat from the dryer gets absorbed into the stagnant water. When the processor is running, the excess heat is flowed out because of the water volume.

Stainless steel is a metal that exists in an active state of controlled oxidation that prevents it from oxidizing in the usual manner called rusting. The steel gives off heavy metal ions that tend to inhibit the growth of algae and bacteria. Plastic and rubberized tanks do not have this feature, so they give the appearance of being prone to growth, especially bio-slime.

The easiest method to combat algae and bio-slime is to make the wash tank self-draining. The tank is always slightly open, so about a quarter of a gallon of water flows out the bottom at all times. Whenever the water flow is turned off, the moisture, food, and warmth, along with any spores and cells, drain out of the tank. The dry tank will not support growth. The open bottom drain will not otherwise affect washing or require a change in volume.

The next step, if needed, is to add a few milliliters (ounces) of liquid laundry bleach (5% sodium hypochlorite) to the wash tank at shutdown. Begin with treatment on Friday nights or Saturday nights. If needed, increase to two or three times per week. If the problem still seems to persist, treat the water at the end of each workday.

The next phase is continuous treatment, which again should begin with a simple system rather than an expensive, complicated approach. For instance, in plastic tanks a sheet of clean copper can be placed in the bottom. The slightly acidic water will erode copper ions, which are a heavy metal. These types of ions inhibit growth of the algae spores and bacteria cells. Tablets, flakes, and dispensers used for purifying swimming pools can be adopted. Liquid laundry bleach, which is inexpensive, can be made into a simple continuous-feed system by adding a small replenishment pump. The pump can be tied to the processor's film detection switch or can be controlled by a timer. A simple dispenser can be made from a piece of rigid polyvinyl-chloride pipe with holes drilled in it and the ends capped.

One of the problems with dispensers is that they have a tendency to run out. If they are empty, they stop working.

Commercial continuous-treatment devices such as chlorine gas injection, water halogenation plants, and ultraviolet light treatment are available.

Wetting Agent

Function

Wetting agents are used primarily in manual processing but occasionally in cine processors. The function of this chemical bath is to allow water from the wash stages to flow off the film more easily. It is said that a wetting agent makes water wetter. Water is a dry chemical in that it has a high surface tension and thus beads up easily. Should a bead or droplet of water dry on a film, the minerals contained would be formed into crystals and would leave disturbing marks. Thus, the wetting agent is used. It lowers the surface tension of water so that it flows off a film rather than beading. A film needs to be in the wetting agent for only a second or two. Modern processors do not need the wetting agent because of the shorter wash time, less gelatin in the emulsion, harder gelatin, processor squeegee action, and the use of a developer hardener.

Types

All wetting agents reduce the water surface tension so that the water flows off the film, thus they are similar. Photo-flo is a longtime favorite of photographers. Dupanol by Du Pont is another brand. Should a wetting agent be needed, they are commonly purchased at photographic supply stores. A pharmacist can also supply general wetting agents based on hexametaphospate.

Archival Quality

Documents of archival quality by definition remain unchanged for a period of time. Long-term patient films must usually be stored for 5 years, according to general agreement among the medical community and also by law in areas such as New York State and Canada. Some federal and military groups require that films be kept for longer periods of time, possibly the life of the patient. Some industrial requirements are 40 years after death, separation, or retirement. The purpose of keeping patient films for a period of time obviously is to afford the radiologist or researcher reviewing a history to better understand a patient's or worker's health and medical evolution. However, it is not sufficient simply to "store" patient films. The key word in the definition is *unchanged*. Should the films become scratched, wet, or stained, information may be altered. The most common problem is stain. Thiosulfate from the fixer clearing agent left in the film after washing can react with silver, producing Ag_2S. This compound produces a stain that ranges from pale yellow to dark amber or brown. The pale yellow is initially combined with the blue tint of the film base to produce a green color similar to unprocessed film except that it is transparent. Any amount of stain, in effect, voids the ability to read the film (Fig. 5-5).

In a legal case, the stained film could be judged to be an alteration of evidence, possibly negating its value. Once the stain is formed, it is difficult to remove and even more difficult to prevent production of a worse condition subsequently. Usually, when poor archival quality is encountered, the wash water is suspected as not having been warm enough or of insufficient flow (agitation). More often, too much fixer is left in the film, causing stain because of a weak developer hardener and/or weak fixer. Finally, and most important, is the consideration of film storage conditions. No matter how well a film is washed, any amount of thiosulfate and silver left in the film can react under the proper conditions. All chemical reactions are controlled by elements of time, temperature, and activity. In this case, time is dictated. However, long-term films are often relegated to such unused areas as the basement, next to the boiler. The resulting high temperature and humidity will initiate the reaction. Thus, regardless of the residual hypo (retained thiosulfate), it is critical that films be stored at 23°C (70°F) and 60% relative humidity (RH) or lower. The basic formula would be as follows:

$$S_2O_3^- \quad + \quad Ag^+ \rightarrow \text{time (fixed)} \quad \rightarrow \quad Ag_2S$$

$$\text{Thiosulfate} \quad \text{Silver} \quad \text{temperature} \quad \text{Silver sulfide}$$
$$\text{activity} (H_2O) \quad \text{(stain)}$$

Measurement

There are two methods used to measure the potential archival quality or amount of residual thiosulfate (hypo retained). The first is an estimator (e.g., Eastman Kodak Hypo Estimator), which requires a drop of silver nitrate

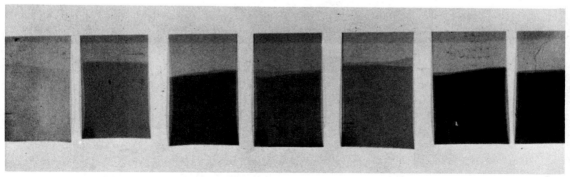

Fig. 5-5.   Stain affecting the archival quality of film.

to be placed on the film. After 15 seconds, the amount of stain produced is compared with various test patches to determine the level of acceptability. This system is often used in industrial radiography and general photography. It is limited because it considers only untinted, single-emulsion films. Thus to use it for radiography, accurately, is very difficult. Remember to double the value determined because of the two emulsion layers. Keep in mind that this is only an estimator, as the name states. It is available from photographic supply stores.

The second method is that recommended by ANSI in their document PH 1.41, 1976. This details an analytical method by which a piece of film is treated in several chemicals to force the appearance of the silver sulfide stain. The dried film is then read on a densitometer using a filter wheel. A blue filter is required because of the yellow stain. The measurement derived is in micrograms per square centimeter (μg/cm^2) or micrograms per square inch (μg/inch^2). This is called the densitometric method. It is a practical approach based on the more difficult methylene blue analytical procedure. Most film companies offer hypo retention testing.

Levels of Acceptability

The ANSI level is 8 μg/cm^2 (24 μg/inch^2), but that is not a hard and fast rule or a guarantee. For instance, a level of 5 to 8 μg/cm^2 of residual thiosulfate left in a film stored next to a boiler at 32°C (90°F) and 90% RH or higher will probably stain much sooner than the prescribed 5 years and also sooner than, for example, a film at a level of 25 μg/cm^2 stored at 5°C (40°F) and 40% RH. Remember that storage conditions play a significant role in the chemical reaction.

Typically, it is expected that a warm-water processor with good developer, fixer, and adequate wash would produce level of 0 to 2 μg/cm^2 (0 to 10 μg/inch^2). A cold-water processor would produce 4 to 8 μg/cm^2. Since cold water means 0°C (32°F) to 32°C (90°F), it is very important to perform a hypo retention test in a cold-water processor in the coldest part of winter and the warmest part of summer. Storage conditions must either be adjusted to the worst condition or the water must be warmed up.

Several film manufacturers provide free analysis based on the ANSI standard. This requires that an unexposed 8 × 10 film from the film bin be normally processed. The film should represent everyday, usual film of good quality. Record all processing conditions. Identify processor, location, date, etc. Submit the processed film to your local technical representative for analysis. The resulting Hypo retention report or archival quality analysis provides an excellent aid to making decisions about how to improve the processing. This report also is a significant document for your quality control program.

Chemical Causes and Remedies

Developer hardener failure allows the gelatin to swell excessively and to absorb too much developer. This, in turn, will result in excess fixer pickup. The fixer and wash cycles are set to accomplish certain tasks in a fixed time frame. The excess swelling and subsequent fixer pickup cannot be compensated for by either the fixer hardener or the water. The water cannot dilute out the excess fixer in the time provided. The result is reduced archival quality as a result of excess fixer (hypo retention, residual thiosulfate).

To determine developer hardener failure is difficult, so the only recourse is to perform a fixer clearing time test to ensure that the fixer is correctly functioning. This is faster and easier than changing the developer solution. When changing the developer, do not refill from the replenishment tank unless the replenisher chemical is relatively fresh. This is because the replenisher may be weak. If the volume of replenisher is low, throw it away and make a fresh batch.

Excessively high pH, overdilution, abnormally high temperature, and poor squeegee roller action can all contribute to excess gelatin swelling in the developer, but these are less common causes. Fixer temperature is a passive system in that it often is not controlled and simply accumulates heat throughout the workday. Should the fixer temperature exceed the developer temperature, the gelatin will override the hardener's ability to control swelling. The excess fixer will not be washed out, since the wash cycle cannot compensate. The pH and dilution also affect gelatin swell and fixer absorption. Hypo retention stain is caused by Ag_2S, which is formed by a reaction of the fixer's thiosulfate and silver. When the fixer dissolves out the silver halide crystals, a complex compound of silver-thiosulfate is formed and is easily converted to Ag_2S. Sodium sulfite, the fixer preservative, normally dissolves the silver out of the complex and regenerates the thiosulfate. Thus, sodium sulfite is very important to controlling Ag_2S stain. It is destroyed by an electrolysis in a recirculating silver recovery cell. It is depleted by overdilution, incorrect mixing, or underreplenishment. An indication of preservative (sulfite) failure is increased clearing time. Usually, when there is a high hypo retention level, the wash water is immediately suspected. As noted above, the water can only function within its time/temperature/agitation frame. If the film product is improperly treated prior to the wash, the wash cannot compensate. The usual water problem is lack of warmth or lack of agitation. The colder the water, the lower the washing (dilution) efficiency. Lower agitation also reduces efficiency. In cold-water processors, the water volume is usually about 4 L (1 gallon) per minute. In some parts of the country, the cold water might approach 0°C (32°F) in the coldest part of the winter. Thus it is very important to perform a hypo retention test in the warmest part of the summer and the coldest part of winter. If the water is too cold, it must be warmed up, which is best accomplished by using a mixing valve. If the water flow volume is too high, lower it to save warm water. If the volume is at 4 L or less, consider installing a recirculation pump to increase the agitation. A basic recommendation would be to install a mixing valve on all cold-water processor. If the water needs to be warmed up, the mixing valve permits warm water to be blended in. Cold water may only have to be raised 5 to 10°. High-recovery water heaters or demand heaters are also recommended.

Storage Conditions

Regardless of the residual thiosulfate retained in film, the storage conditions are critical. All chemical reactions are initiated or controlled by elements of time, temperature, and activity. For archival quality, the reaction of thiosulfate and silver to produce silver sulfide is controlled by temperature and relative humidity. The higher the temperature and/or humidity, the shorter is the storage time. For archival purposes, the general rule is to store films at 20°C (68°F) or less and at 60% RH or less.

The films must not be stored in the boiler room, where it is very hot and humid, because even an acceptably washed film (less than 8 $\mu g/cm^2$) can stain more quickly than usual. The easiest method of controlling heat is to install a basic air-conditioner unit in a designated storage room. Since the heat factors are static inside the room, not much capacity is needed to maintain temperature.

The same air-conditioner will also control humidity. However, because of fumes and moisture from the films, an air agitation-airflow-ventilation arrangement is advised. If a room is adequately cooled without need for additional cooling, then only forced ventilation is required to move out fumes and keep the air fresh.

Summary and Conclusion

Processing completes what the exposure started. Development selectively converts the latent image into the useful visible image with amplification of about 10^9 times. Fixer removes undeveloped crystals. The wash removes the fixer to permit long-term storage (archival quality).

Processing is a chemical process (development, fixation, washing) that is controlled by elements of time (immersion in solution), temperature, and activity (chemical brand and type, replenishment, agitation). The pH, specific gravity, mixing procedures, and hardener levels all influence chemical efficiency.

Should processing be inferior (less than optimal), then the best technology available for producing the latent image will be lost because an inferior visible image will be produced. Processing directly affects image quality. It is beneficial to the modern radiology department to have a processing specialist or quality control technologist on staff who is knowledgeable in this area of chemistry and processing.

Chapter 6

The Electromechanical Systems

In processing, the basic chemical reactions are controlled by elements of time, temperature, and activity. In manual processing, these same functions are primarily controlled by hand. *Time* is time in solution, which is a function of transport and thus is called the transport system. Temperature must be controlled, and thus the temperature control or tempering system. Activity includes replacing lost chemical volume (replenishment) and replacing consumed chemicals to sustain strength (regeneration), thus, a replenishment/regeneration system. Activity also includes agitation to provide uniform chemicals (strength and temperature) and completeness of function. Agitation is one of four functions of the circulation/filtration system. Of course, activity includes the chemistry system, which was discussed in the previous chapter and is not an electromechanical system. The dryer system dries the film for convenience and to help preserve the image. Electricity is used in each of the five systems listed above, constituting an electrical system. The six electromechanical systems support the chemical reactions. These systems in an automatic processor are only quasi-automatic or semiautomatic. They require adjustment, control, monitoring, and service by an operator. Indeed, an automatic processor in radiography is not truly automatic since it does not monitor film quality and adjust itself to produce consistent quality.

Transport System

Function

The transport system should move or convey the film through the various chemicals at the correct speed without damage (Fig. 6-1). It handles the film by means of the rollers in the conveyor subsystem and moves the film from point to point at a certain speed by means of gears, sprockets, and/or chains (drive subsystem) (Fig. 6-2).

Components

The conveyor subsystem is composed of the feed tray, crossover rollers (or roller assemblies), deep racks with their turnaround assemblies, and receiver bin. The rollers range in composition from hard to soft and in size from approximately 0.6 cm (¼ inch) to 7.6 cm (3 inches). Racks of rollers are held in alignment by faceplates and tie bars. Usually, film direction is changed by deflector plates or guide shoes.

The drive subsystem (Fig. 6-3) starts with a gear motor that drives a sprocket, which then drives a chain, or a gear that drives another gear. This energy drives the main drive shaft, which in turn drives the individual racks and ultimately the individual rollers. All of the rollers should turn at the same speed.

film path

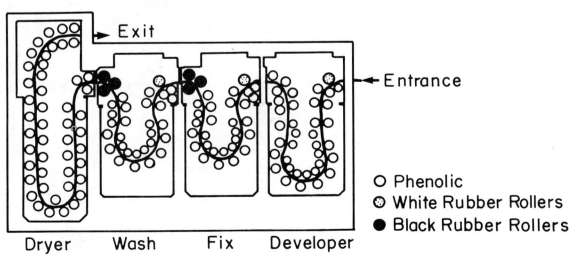

Fig. 6-1.   Transport system.

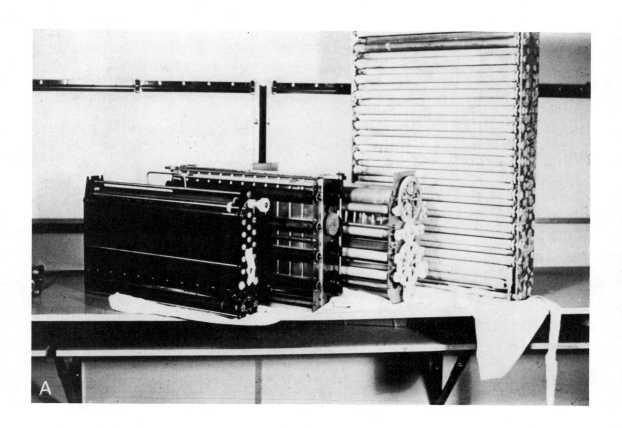

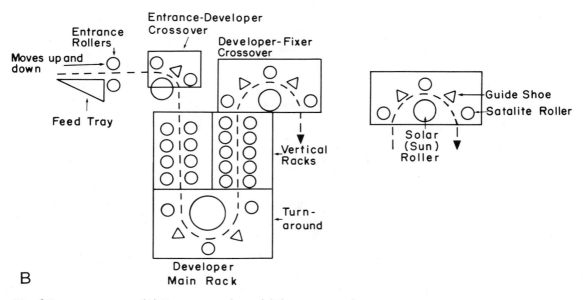

Fig. 6-2.   (A) Transport racks and (B) conveyor subsystem.

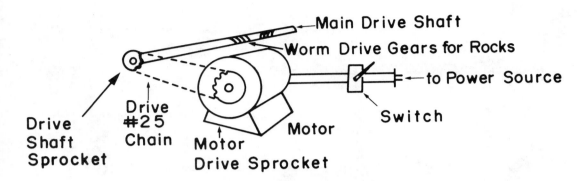

Fig. 6-3.   Drive subsystem.

Feed Tray

The feed tray aligns the film for proper transport. Along the outside edges there are rails or raised edges for guiding the film. These should always be used. The tray is polished, but not to the extent that it will not produce scratches. Thus, fingers must be placed behind the trailing edge of the film to push it into the entrance detector crossover or assembly rather than placed on top of the film. The feed tray is usually supported by a support box or a shelf. The box and the tray are adjustable in position (up and down) and tilt (left to right and front to back). Adjust the tray so that film being fed strikes the upper quadrant (quarter) of the lower entrance roller. This helps ensure that the film is lifted off the entrance edge of the tray, which often gets dirty and is somewhat difficult to clean. Daily cleaning with a mild soap solution and a soft rag is required. If the environment in the darkroom is unusually dusty, increase cleaning frequency and/or keep the tray covered during slack times. Disconnect the feed tray weekly to clean the leading edge. Note that on most Eastman Kodak processors the feed tray can swivel in the direction of film travel and is adjustable by three wing nuts under the feed tray support box. Alignment is important and should be checked periodically.

Conveyor Subsystem

The rollers that handle the film range from hard to soft. The hardest are Plexiglas and stainless steel. These rollers are easy to clean, but if they become dirty or damaged they will expose the film with a pressure mark (this will be visible only if prior to fixation). Next in degree of hardness are polyester, polyethylene, and polypropylene rollers. Phenolic is the oldest roller material and is still in use today. These rollers are made of phenol resin and cellulose and appear as orange-brown "wooden" rollers. They are somewhat porous, and excessive or harsh cleaning with abrasive pads will wear down the material. Placing these rollers in acid solutions (fixer, systems cleaners) will draw out the solvents, resulting in gas pockets. These pockets will heave up the surface material, producing wet pressure sensitization in the developer rack and developer-to-fixer crossover. Soft rollers have a synthetic covering of elastic-plastic or elastomer on a harder core. A thin layer or sleeve might be on a large steel core or on top of sponge. A thinner material is more prone to deterioration than a thicker layer. Sponge can be open pore or closed pore. Open-pore sponge has a rough or broken-bubble surface, which promotes chemical activity. Closed-pore sponge does not have broken bubbles. Open-pore sponge cannot be cleaned if it becomes dirty or contaminated. Sponge rollers offer a much reduced chance of pressure marks, since the material is resilient. All of these soft rollers are referred to as resilient rollers, and they must have a hard steel core to help maintain shape or roundness.

Pi marks were first recognized only as pi lines. A roller in an older processor, with older-style thicker emulsions, would pick up a line of gelatin from chipping of the leading edge of the film. This line of gelatin would be carried around the circumference of a roller and deposited back onto the film. The roller usually was 2.54 cm (1 inch) in diameter, so the redeposited line occurred 8 cm (3.14 inches) in from the leading edge. Since 3.14 is the mathematical constant referred to as pi, (Greek symbol π), this line of gelatin particles was called a pi line. Today the line problem is not as prevalent as repeating marks such as wet pressure sensitization. The circumference of a roller is 3.14 times the diameter. Most rollers are 2.54 cm (1 inch) in diameter, although they range from 1.9 to 7.6 cm (¾ to 3 inches) in diameter. A mark repeating every 8 cm (3.14 or 3⅛ inches) would be caused by a 2.54-cm (1-inch) diameter roller; 16 cm (6.28 or 6¼ inches) repeating patterns are caused by a 5.08-cm (2-inch) roller. Remember that plus-density (black) marks must occur prior to fixation.

Crossovers (see Fig. 6-2B) carry the film from one stage to the next and cross over the partition between stages, thus their name. The various crossover units are entrance (or entrance detector if film sensors are included)-to-developer, developer-to-fixer, fixer-to-wash, and wash-to-dryer (or exit, or exit squeegee). Crossovers may be separate, removable racks consisting of two or more rollers or may be a part of the vertical rack assembly. Crossover rollers are out of solution, so that chemicals carried onto them by the passage of film can dry out and become sticky or crystalline and sharp. It is important to use fume control hoods (small covers) to keep the chemicals from drying out. Also, crossovers and all rollers out of solution must be cleaned prior to processing work films. If the processor is on standby for longer than 2 hours, the crossovers should be recleaned. Opening the processor lid and removing fume hoods at the end of a workday help to let moisture escape. Crossovers as separate components tend to twist easily and become misaligned.

Turnarounds are components found at the bottom of a vertical rack assembly. Their function is to turn the film around from a downward movement to an upward movement. They could be a series of 2.54-cm (1-inch) rollers making a tight conveyor path or a pivotal roller with smaller rollers and guide shoes. In the latter case, the pivotal roller is usually 5.08 cm (2 inches) in diameter, such as in typical Eastman Kodak X-OMAT M5 to M6-AW processors. To the outside of the center pivotal roller (called a B roller by Kodak) are two spring-loaded 2.54-cm (1-inch) resistant rollers designated A rollers. The entire assembly is an adjustable member that places tension on the ladder-style drive chain (Fig. 6-4). Great care is required to ensure that all corners of the floating turnaround are spaced equally. The vertical rack places very little stress on the film, and thus few problems occur here. It is basically a box composed of rollers, tie bars, and faceplates (end plates). The roller configuration might be staggered, as originally developed by Kodak; opposing, as typical of Pako, AFP, and others; or slightly staggered, such as in Hope

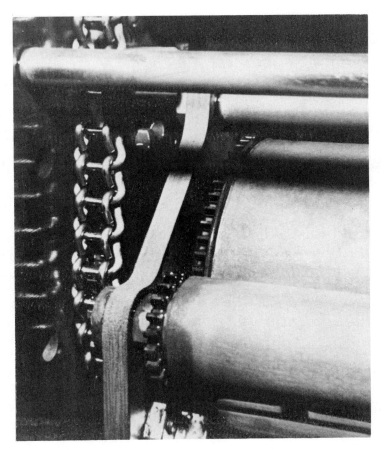

Fig. 6-4.   Ladder chain.

products (Profexray Litton, Du Pont). The staggered rollers place very little pressure on the film and thus are more prone to transport problems. Opposing rollers offer a more positive pressure system, but a small pile of dirt (gelatin) can cause a film mark. Thus there basically is no single perfect rack design, since each has strong points and weak points. The preferred transport system would be rollerless.

Guide shoes are also called deflector plates. They direct the film in those places where the film might choose its own path as a result of inherent curl, roller pressure, or pressure from the circulation pump. In a vertical rack assembly, films tend to curl one way between widely spaced rollers and the deflector plates (which may be fingers or wire bars) deflect the film back into the next roller set. At crossovers and turnarounds where the film is being changed in direction, it is important to remember that the film has a thick (7 mils) plastic base that has a memory. It wants to lie flat. Thus, the guide shoe directs the film around the corner. In turnarounds, there are either two guide shoes and three rollers or three guide shoes and two rollers. Crossovers usually have two rollers and two shoes. Fixed guide shoes are usually removable for cleaning and might become bent, so they should be inspected. There is no adjustment included. However, should a persistent problem develop, such as scratches, the plate can be reshaped or the mounting holes changed slightly. Adjustable guide shoes are less secure and require periodic readjustment. Guide shoe "finger" (long protrusions) scratches should be uniform and never more than 0.6 cm (0.25 inches) long. The guide shoe entrance should be wide open to catch film, and the exit should be closed down to feed the film into the next roller pinch (impingement) point. After adjusting, run a wet green film through the racks (on a bench, not in the processor) and check for scratches. If scratches appear, then a guide shoe is too tight. Adjustable guide shoes usually are only found in Kodak processors. The shoe has slots that allow sideways movement of the shoe to help in determining which shoe is causing scratches. Allen or pan-head screws attach and hold the shoe to the adjustable mounting blocks. Any type of shoe must be inspected for alignment relative to nearby rollers. Guide shoes sometimes have protrusions called fingers. The longer fingers usually point in the direction the film is going. The shorter fingers, or the edge without fingers, or the rounded-off edge is usually the trailing edge, since the trailing edge of the film usually hits against it. If there are no fingers on either edge or if they are of equal length, then observe the support brace position. It tends to be toward the entrance side of the shoe. The front of the guide shoe would then be the longer feed end. Side plates or faceplates might be fiberboard, stainless steel, or plastic. When these plates are pulled tight by tie bars, they form a box to hold and align the roller conveyor assembly. It is important to inspect the faceplates for wear and squareness. All types of material will eventually wear away or fatigue. Tie bars work with the side plates. They usually are stainless steel, whereas their nuts might be steel or plastic and the side plates might be fiberboard, steel, or plastic. With temperature rise and fall, these dissimilar materials expand and contract at different rates, causing the components to loosen. When a rack assembly (plates and tie bars) is loose, it can twist out of alignment, causing transport problems. Misalignment often occurs when the rack is removed from or replaced into the processor.

Racks are driven by chains and sprockets and/or gears. Since the main drive force enters the rack only on one side, a large force is applied to only one point or side—torque. Torque is work being applied. It is important to transmit this torque to the opposite end of the rack so that it turns with and does not lag behind the drive side. This is called torque balance or distribution. A poorly balanced rack will become twisted and result in transport problems.

Eastman Kodak racks are driven by means of a ladder chain and sprockets, which in turn drive gears (see Fig. 6-4). Sprockets run on chains. The ladder chain is more correctly termed wire chain, since it consists of hooks and bars made from wire. There is no master link; any link can be opened to break the chain. When opening the link, try to rotate the loop open rather than straighten out the loop. The tension on the chain is achieved by moving the adjustable turnaround assembly. Never make the chain as tight as you can, since this accentuates wearing. Light tension and frequent inspection are all that is needed. One way to gauge tightness is to grasp one or two rollers in the vertical section, turn the main drive gear, and see if the chain slips, which would indicate that the chain was too loose. The chain should be positioned so that the loop pulls down on the bar and faces outward. It is possible to install the chain upside down and/or backward. When inside out, the loop can deteriorate sprockets. When upside down, the chain tends to stretch because the loops open up. The steel wire will wear in several areas.

Gears operate or run against other gears. They must be in alignment and mesh properly but not excessively. Also, the rollers and the gears should have some degree of freedom since they are cast from plastic rather than machined from steel. Plastics will swell in chemical solution. Dissimilar plastics can swell up and jam a rack. Inspect the gears at least monthly for signs of wear. Check tightness when they are warm and emerging directly from the chemical bath.

Racks are supported by a support bar. Kodak racks hang from two external bearings surrounding the main rack drive shaft. These bearings must not turn with the shaft. The bearings sit in support bars. These bars or their support pedestals are often adjustable. The drive side support bar near the main drive motor usually is the only point to get out of adjustment. Periodic critical testing with a level is all that is needed. Pako, Du Pont, and Picker racks hang by hooks or ledges on three and four points. Hope-built processors generally have the rack sitting on the bottom of the chemical tank rather than hanging. If the main processor drive train consists of worm gears on a shaft, it is important that no weight be placed on the shaft because this could warp and destroy the bearings, motor, or gears. If the drivetrain is a flat gear train, then the gears must not be elevated to the point where they cause lifting and/or tilting of the rack.

Drive Subsystem

Figure 6-3 is a diagram of the drive subsystem. The main drive motor is less than 1 hp and, thus, is listed as fractional horsepower. Most manufacturers use $\frac{1}{8}$ to $\frac{1}{20}$ hp, and one manufacturer uses $\frac{1}{20}$ to $\frac{1}{90}$ hp. The larger the fraction, the smaller the unit is: $\frac{1}{90}$ hp is not quite half as big as $\frac{1}{50}$ hp. These small motors run on less than 1 A.

To start the motor and to overcome the weight of all of the rollers and transport system is quite a task. One method is to use a condenser (often called a can since it is shaped like an oval can), which builds 115 volts of alternating current (VAC) up to 320 VAC. This large voltage moves the rotor into position to become synchronized with alternating current. Some motors are condenser run; they build up current and fire or discharge continually. Split-phase starting uses a second bundle of wire (start windings) that consists of finer wire and less of it than the windings that function when the motor is running. When an electrical current is passed through both bundles, a phase shift of electromotive force is created. That is, magnetic pull is exerted sequentially in one and then the other winding. The rotor starts to turn and becomes synchronized with the alternating current in the running windings. The starter windings must be turned off within a second or two to prevent them from burning out. This is accomplished by a centrifugal throw-out switch mounted on the nondrive end of the rotor.

Motors having starting windings are labeled universal/reversible, since the motor can be run in either direction by changing the sequence of electromotive impulses between start and run windings. The start windings are always blue wires, and the run windings are always black wires. One combination of black and blue leads tied together and connected to a power source, such as L1, will drive the motor in one direction when the other black and blue wires are attached to the appropriate line (L2 or N). Changing the blue wire attached to a black will reverse the direction.

These motors run at 1725 to 1750 rpm, which is too fast. Thus they usually have a gear reduction mechanism to reduce the speed to 10 to 20 rpm. Each gearbox contains one gear that will break easily in the event of an overload. Gears and gear ratios are replaceable separately from the motor. Indeed, the motor's output shaft is really the gearbox drive shaft and not the drive shaft of the motor's rotor. Gear ratios run in 30–60–90 or 20–40–60–80 jumps. A parallel motor is mounted parallel to the processor's drive shaft. The gearbox is in parallel. A right angle or perpendicular motor is one with a vertical motor perpendicular to the processor drive shaft. The gearbox makes a right-angle turn so that its shaft is parallel to the processor's main drive shaft.

Fixed motors run at one speed, whereas adjustable motors offer a variety of speeds. The fixed motor runs on alternating current (AC). The adjustable motor requires a rectifier that converts the AC into DC (direct current). A potentiometer then restricts the amount of current so the motor runs more slowly. Since this system is more expensive and inherently less accurate or stable, it should be avoided. If it is installed, a tachometer must also be installed. DC motors have brushes and a commutator. Adjustable motors are often incorrectly termed variable motors. Adjustable drives built into a processor are more stable than add-on adjustable drives.

Motors are composed of an iron core rotor inside stator windings. These windings include run windings along with start windings and are housed in the center frame, which has a specification tag affixed to the outside. On one end of the unit there is a end bell, which contains a bearing assembly to support the rotor and a start cutout switch. The opposite end is composed of the gear reduction end bell. In perpendicular motors there is usually a gear reduction end bell support. Gear reduction is in odd or even units, such as 20–40–60:1 or 30–60–90:1. Most are 90:1. A gearbox assembly for a motor frame type NSH-12RG will fit on any other NSH-12RG but not on an NSI-11D3A or different motor frame.

Stator windings are composed of run windings and start windings. Both bundles are separate from each other. A bundle is a continuous line of wire with a thin insulation coating of varnish. The start windings generally are smaller, use smaller-diameter wire, and are placed between the run bundles. When a motor fails to start immediately because of excess load, misalignment, or lack of lubrication, the switch must be turned off immediately to prevent damage to the start windings. When a motor fails to start, it usually is because of burned-out start windings. Such motors can be manually started by advancing the cooling fan in the motor using an insulated screwdriver.

As mentioned above, on the motor's center frame a specification tag will list motor frame type, manufacturer's reference number, and other data such as horsepower, amperage, voltage, torque, gear ratio, and both motor and output shaft revolutions per minute. Degrees temperature rise (°C temp rise) indicates how hot the motor can get before the insulation breaks down and the unit shorts out. This is often about 50°C (122°F), which is quite warm.

Gears used to convey energy from the main drive motor to the processor drive shaft or drivetrain are usually designated 16Y12 or Y1612. The 16 refers to the diametral pitch of the teeth as 16° angle. The Y alpha code and its positions are unimportant. The last group of numbers is the number of teeth, in this case 12 teeth. Gears have from 10 to 200 teeth. The drive shaft openings are usually 1.27 to 1.59 cm (½ or ⅝ inches). In Hope-built processors, the main drive gear is held in place by a tapered spleen that is drawn tight by bolts threaded into the gear. Removing these bolts and placing them in threaded spleen flange holes and pushing against the gear results in a self-extracting mechanism. A gear puller only makes the unit tighter and cannot be used. A sandwich pack of two plates and idler gears keeps the main drive gear lined up in contact with the driven gear. The plastic gears of the drivetrain should be loose and wobbly, and if they are adjustable, they should only engage the tips of the gears. To reduce plastic-to-plastic friction, which produces jogging (erratic turning), apply a light coat of grease to all gears outside of the solutions.

Sprockets run on chain. The main drive chain is a number 25 chain, which runs on a number 25 sprocket. The *2* means that the diametral pitch of the teeth is ⅜-inch or ¼-inch pitch. The *5* means that this is nonroller roller chain, and each link joint bends on a pin and sleeve. Roller chain has a separate roller or sleeve bearing around the joint. The chain in processors lacks this roller. Sprockets sizes range from K2512 to 25B48. The second number set is the number of teeth. The alpha code and its position are unimportant. The shaft sizes are 1.27 or 1.59 cm (½ or ⅝ inches), with a 0.95-cm (⅜ inch) shaft in EK M-7 units. A key is often used to lock the sprocket against the shaft. A setscrew secures the lateral movement. Sprockets are not case hardened, but the chain is case hardened, so when there is misalignment or lack of lubrication the sprocket will wear. Frequent inspection and adjustment are called for. Chains should have only 0.6 cm (¼ inch) deflection by gravity at the midpoint between the main drive and driven sprockets. Alignment is best accomplished by looking to see if the sprocket teeth are in the center of the chain link or to one side. Inspect on top and bottom of various sprockets.

Gears out of solution can be coated lightly with grease. Sprockets and chains out of solution require a light coating of light oil. In both cases, remove excess lubricants and periodically remove oxidized lubricants prior to re-lubricating. Avoid getting petroleum products in the chemical tanks or on rollers. Gears and the processor main drive shaft near chemicals can be cleaned and lubricated with a glycerin and water solutions. Use a small, stiff paintbrush to apply.

The dryer drive is often a drive belt/gear arrangement but may use only gears. Inspect tension and belt alignment when the unit is hot, not cold. Test for transport characteristics by running a wet film through the hot dryer and not a dry film through a cool dryer. Never make the drive belt as tight as possible, since this accentuates wear. The tension device is at the bottom turnaround pully, usually in all Kodak units except M7 and M8. If the drive mechanism involves gears, then the dryer is usually a separate rack assembly. Make certain that the rack is square and is properly installed prior to adjusting gear alignment and tension, which should be done when the unit is hot, not cool. Because of the dryer blower, lubricants must be avoided. However, removing friction-causing dirt is a form of lubrication.

Temperature Control System

Function

It is the function of the temperature control system to control the temperature of each of the components in the chemistry system (development, fixation, washing) and the dryer. Of these, controlling the developer temperature is most important. In addition to heating the solutions (and dryer), this system must also compensate for the high ambient conditions inside the processor cabinet and outside, surrounding the processor in the light room and darkroom.

Components

Development temperature control is by means of a thermocouple or heating element controlled by a thermostat and a heat exchanger. Stainless steel tank walls convect heat and help stabilize the temperature. Thermometers are mounted in the heat exchanger or a separate box, referred to by Kodak as a thermowell. Electronic devices help control the current to the heaters.

Fixer is usually heated by convection through the stainless steel tank walls. With plastic tanks and cold-water processors, warm developer is often circulated through a heat exchanger in the base of the fixer tank. In older Pakos, warm water was passed through false bottoms and sides of the fixer tank. Seldom is the fixer actively and positively temperature controlled, but this may be more frequent in the future.

Wash water temperature is controlled by an external mixing valve that automatically blends hot and cold water to meet a desired level. In newer cold-water processors, either there is no control or there is some minor heating involving heat exchangers and the warmer developer and/or heat from the dryer. The dryer is controlled by a thermostat that turns on and off one to three heater elements.

Thermostat versus Thermometer

Both the thermostat and thermometer have a gas-filled sensing bulb. Often the gas is ether. As temperature rises, the ether expands and moves down a small tube. The pressure increases until work is performed. In a thermostat, the pressure pushes on a switch that opens, cutting the electrical flow to the heater. Thus thermostats regulate heat or the heater. The position at which the switch opens is controlled by the adjustment knob (screw post), which must be calibrated. In the thermometer, the pressure pushes a needle to indicate the level of heat. Thermometers must be tested to determine if they are working and if they are accurate. All thermometers can be calibrated.

Calibration

As is implied above, it takes some time for the pressure to rise to the point where work can be performed. This is called lag time in response. Thus, when calibrating thermostats and thermometers it is important to allow for lag time in response.

Obtain a known, calibrated test thermometer. Never use glass thermometers filled with mercury or iodine since, should they break, the chemicals pose a hazard to personnel and/or the developer. If the thermometer is not calibrated, test it in the laboratory or by placing it in boiling water (changes with altitude) and ice water. Most hospital laboratories have a standard calibration procedure and/or a master thermometer calibrated by the National Bureau of Standards. Place the test thermometer in the solution tank and allow it to remain for 1 to 5 minutes to reach a stable temperature. Compare the measured temperature to that on the thermostat or thermometer. If there is error on the thermostat, see if the knob has a recessed screw that can be used to adjust the knob position. If the knob is a friction fit and is not adjustable, then change the markings. Thermometers are calibrated by carefully prying off or unscrewing the front bezel trim that holds the glass. In Hope-built processors, a clamp is removed and the whole thermometer is removed. Under a yellow piece of tape will be found the calibration screws. In other units, the pointer is held with two fingers or a small screwdriver as the pointer is moved to the correct position. Push on the thicker portion of the pointer. Recheck the test thermometer. Replace the lens and trim piece. Recheck the test thermometer. There is a lag on heat rise response and on heat loss response, so this becomes a simple and yet time-consuming procedure.

Mixing Valves

Mixing valves are used on warm-water processors to blend hot and cold water to a certain temperature and volume (Fig. 6-5). They automatically control these functions after being set. It is advisable to install mixing valves on all cold-water processors as well. Hot water enters via a volume control valve and strainer on the left side and to the rear at the base of the valve. Cold water enters from the right to the center of the valve. As the temperature rises, the ether-filled coils expand and close off the hot water supply; as the temperature falls, the coils contract and let in more hot water and less cold. The component that moves with temperature changes is called a thermostatic motor. The valve requires at least annual service and rebuilding. Filters of about 5 to 10 μm are used on the supply lines to protect the valve parts. A tempered water shutoff valve after the valve should be used for on/off control rather than the valve itself.

There are often complaints about hot water passing through mixing valves into the heat exchanger (Fig. 6-6), where the hot water overheats the

The Mixing Valve

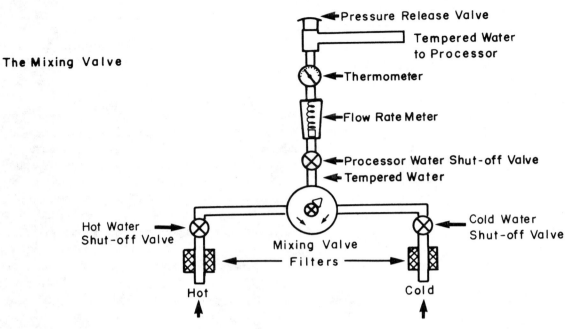

Fig. 6-5.   Tempering system.

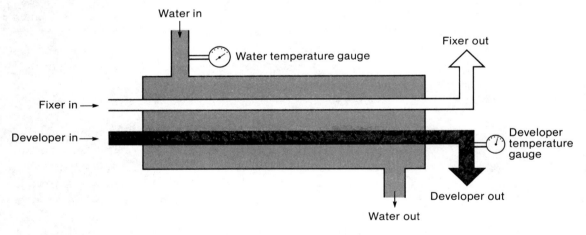

Fig. 6-6.   Heat exchanger.

developer. In a properly adjusted and maintained valve, this phenomenon should not occur since the unit is designed "fail-safe to hot." This means that if only hot water is present, the unit turns off the hot water.

In temperature control, the electrical current that generates the heat results in inefficiency called overshoot and undershoot, which are a drifting of temperatures beyond the desired set point. A typical thermostat is accurate

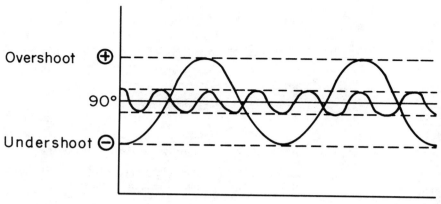

Overshoot ⊕

90°

Undershoot ⊖

Fig. 6-7. Temperature control.

to ± 1°C or F, which is marginal. By using water cooler than the developer and constantly stealing heat through a heat exchanger, the thermostat is made to open and close more rapidly so overshoot and undershoot are reduced to ± ½°C or F (Fig. 6-7). Of course, the greater the temperature difference between the water and the developer, the less the volume; the smaller the temperature difference, the greater the volume of water needed to exchange heat. In cold-water processing, the water may be too cold, so a mixing valve is suggested. The wash water should be warm to wash out chemicals from the gelatin (chemical function) and cool to help control the developer temperature (mechanical function).

To test a mixing valve, simply close off the cold water supply and observe the thermometer. The thermostatic motor should shut down the hot water supply within about 5 seconds and before the thermometer reaches 35°C (95°F). Should the thermometer indicate it will reach higher levels, begin closing down the mixing valve until flow stops. Open the cold water valve and, using volume controls, adjust the temperature and volumes from this point; the mixing valve can be screwed inward but not outward. Be sure to verify that the thermometer is working and accurate before any testing. The thermometer can be calibrated.

Safety Devices

Newer processors with plastic tanks and/or plastic thermowells use thermal cutout safety switches to prevent fires. These units, which are simple thermostats, are usually reset automatically. When they are open, the system shuts down as if broken.

Safety devices are placed over the dryer heater elements. To achieve 55°C (130°F) in the dryer chamber, the heaters are usually closer to 120°C (248°F). The most common safety switch is the Therm-O-Disc brand. Should the disk open the circuit, it will appear that the control thermostat and/or the heaters are broken when they are not. These safety thermostats are usually composed of two metals (bimetallic) of different coefficients of expansion. As they get hot, one metal expands faster than other, causing the strip to bend and opening the circuit. In addition, there might also be electrical protectors such as fuses or circuit breakers.

Motors usually have thermal protection devices to prevent their destruction should they get too hot because of the load or the environment. The motor protector might be located on the motor center frame, screwed to the outside like a top hat, or it might be built into the end bell. The end bell unit is manually resettable. The surface mount automatically resets.

Circulation-Filtration System

Function

There are four functions in the circulation/filtration system: mixing the chemicals for uniform temperature, mixing for uniform activity, agitation, and filtration (Fig. 6-8). In the development stage of the chemical system, the temperature must be exact. Whenever heating or cooling takes place, there must be agitation to provide uniformity and to prevent a small quantity of developer from being oxidized. Replenishment chemicals are cooler and

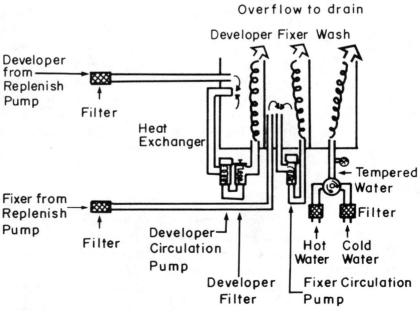

Fig. 6-8.   Circulation system.

stronger (higher pH) and must be rapidly and uniformly blended into the working solution. Debris such as gelatin must be filtered, which requires forcing the solution through a filter. Agitation for the sake of complete chemical reaction is of less importance in the faster processing cycles because the movement of the film through the solution accomplishes the same function. In slower processing cycles, 3 minutes or longer, agitation by a pump contributes to complete development. Not all processors have a developer filter. There is some question about the importance of the developer filter, since many processors have operated for years without filters and without problems. Higher-volume processors need filters primarily because of the increased quantity of debris. Fixer agitation ensures uniform temperature and activity. Again, agitation primarily is provided by the rapid movement of the film through the solution. The clearing action of the fixer is about 10 to 20% more efficient with agitation, but the total fixing time is twice the clearing time. Thus, in an emergency, if only one pump can be made to work, it must be placed on the developer tank.

Wash agitation is primarily supplied by water volume. The water in Profexray-Litton and Du Pont processors is agitated by a recirculation pump. This ensures increased agitation and substantial reduction in water consumption. The pump system can be added to any processor to conserve water. Water filtration serves to protect the mixing valve rather than to supply clean wash water. The smallest particle visible to the unaided eye is 40 μm, but water needs to be filtered to 5 to 10 μm to protect the mixing valve.

Dryer filtration is problematic. Much air is drawn into the blower at a rate of about 200 cubic feet per minute (cfm). A small amount of dirt per hour builds up rapidly. Filtration works very well, except that as it clogs, less air is moved, upsetting the dryer's characteristics. If it is necessary to put in filters, they should be placed so that turbulent air flows past the filters and not through them. Cine processors have air filters that require cleaning daily. Cine processors also have filters on air squeegee devices.

Components

All pumps are assemblies of three parts: electric motor, coupler, and pump head. When a problem occurs, it usually is in the pump head, which is the least expensive component. Most pump assembly designs employ centrifugal magnetic drive. One large magnet on the motor drive shaft turns a smaller impeller magnet inside the plastic pump body. The advantage of this type of pump is that the chemicals never touch the motor or drive components. Chemicals flow into the center of the pump head and are pushed to the outside by the centrifugal force of the impeller.

The plumbing system is composed of flexible polyvinylchloride (PVC) tubing. This tubing is often called Tygon, which is a brand name of the Norton Chemical Company, but other brands are also used. It should have 0.31-cm

(⅛-inch) wall thickness. Tubings of only two or three sizes (inside diameters) are needed. Preformed bends keep the tubing from collapsing in tight areas. Kodak processors usually have line restrictors in the tubing leading away from the pump. The tubing is held tight to fittings by clamps. The clamps should be of the screw type.

Filters are either disposable or nondisposable (cleanable). Chemicals should come to the outside of the filter and pass to the center. A clogged filter can reduce agitation and even burn out pumps. The three most common sources of problems are selecting the incorrect pore size, caking, and channeling. Too large a filter (pore) size allows debris to pass through. Caking results when too small a pore size is used. Channeling results from inexpensive filters, physical damage, and/or excess pressure. A channel passes all the fluid without removing any debris. Filters are rated in micrometers (μm) pore size, but the word *microns* (μ) is also used.

Pumps

Centrifugal magnetic-drive and direct-drive pumps are the two types of pumps used. Both types use centrifugal force to move fluids. All pumps are assemblies of three parts: an electric motor, a coupler, and a pump head. In magnetic-drive pumps, a main drive magnet passes magnetic impulses through the plastic pump head to a driven magnet attached to an impeller. Running the pump dry will cause the impeller to deteriorate. If either magnet abrades on the plastic, a loud screaming sound will result. The drive magnet is held in place with a setscrew that can loosen with time. The two parts of the pump head are held together with wing nuts. An O-ring makes the two halves tight to hold solutions. Should the O-ring be damaged, it can be repaired with silicon glue (bathtub caulk). A large rubber band could also be used to make a compression seal. Direct-drive pumps are also called sump pumps or column pumps. The motor sits on top of a column. Inside the column, attached directly to the motor drive shaft, is a long shaft with an impeller at the end. Near the impeller, in the column, is a bearing. Around the shaft is a bearing surface. These pumps should never be operated without fluid, since the fluid provides lubrication between the two bearing components. When the impeller is dry, it will have a tendency to "whip," causing more rapid deterioration. The impeller shaft is connected by a double screw, a screw and a coupler, or a coupler. A common problem occurs when the inner column becomes locked into the outer housing. Flushing with warm water may help. The next step would be to warm the outer housing and cool the inner column. At the bottom of the column there is an O-ring that should be inspected frequently and replaced before it deteriorates or joins the column and housing together.

Plumbing

Plumbing is referred to as the tubing. The only rigid tubes are water lines. Most tubing is flexible PVC. The developer is drawn from the bottom of the tank, into the filter, into the thermowell to be heated, into the pump, out of the pump through a heat exchanger, and then back into the developer tank. The fixer circuit is very basic. Fixer flows to the pump and back to the tank. Replenishment lines can feed directly into the tank through the side wall or over the top. Excess chemicals overflow a weir (dam) to the common drain. Tanks can have bottom drains or removable standpipes. The important consideration usually is that the pump be mounted below the level of the tank drain. When the tank is drained, a quantity of fluid is left in the circulatory system and pump head. Tank drains could be a simple large tube, a totally closed canister called a header assembly, or an open trough. In all cases, it is important to run water whenever chemicals are drained to help prevent buildup. Flexible tubing should have a wall thickness of 0.31 cm (⅛ inch). This tubing should be replaced annually in pieces or all at once. At that time, replace T's and Y's. A line restrictor is generally a plastic plug placed in the line near the outlet of the pump. An orifice or opening is drilled in the center. This restrictor is placed on the outlet side of the pump and serves to increase velocity but also to reduce flow. As tubing deteriorates or filters clog, the resistance to flow will increase.

Clamps

Spring clamps or hose clamps are slowly being eliminated from use. They are a piece of spring metal formed into a loop or circle. They are inexpensive and designed to be used only once, such as in manufacturing. Their installation and removal require a special pair of pliers that have notches in the heads to grip the clamp tangs (or tires). Regular pliers must not be used because the clamp can slip and literally shoot out, causing damage. When working with these clamps, always wear safety glasses because the clamp can break into several pieces with tremendous force. To remove a clamp, apply the special pliers and move the clamp off the fitting, release the tension on the clamp, remove the tubing from the fitting, and slide the clamp off and discard it. These clamps are often called Corbin clamps, but Corbin is only one manufacturer. Screw clamps are more expensive but are reusable. Select one or two sizes similar to the tubing size found in the processor. One or two turns and the clamp is open; two turns and the clamp is tight.

Plastic snap clamps have recently become more common. These units apparently can be installed with only finger pressure. However, to properly seal tubing to fittings, a pair of pliers must be applied to draw the plastic clamp tighter. The clamp maintains tension by interlocking teeth like a ratchet. To open the clamp, twist or pry the two teeth assemblies apart.

Filters

Filters may be disposable or nondisposable, in-depth or surface effect (Fig. 6-9). Surface filters are a fine mesh of wire or plastic that can be easily cleaned and reused. After washing or before installing, be sure to force water through the mesh to wet the inner faces of the mesh to prevent air block. These types of filters clog more rapidly and are usually found in replenishment lines. Their function is to keep debris from jamming, clogging, or damaging the pump mechanism poppet valves, flow meters, and/or adjustment valves. Strainers, usually found in mixing-valve supply lines, have large pore openings and look like copper window screening although they are sometimes perforated metal. In-depth filters may be thought of as a stack of surface filters. A particle is trapped by one of the layers, and the filter is used until the entire depth is filled with debris. Since the filter wall is very deep (2.54 cm [1 inch]), it cannot be efficiently cleaned so it is made to be discarded. It is difficult to determine when to discard a filter. One way is to weigh it clean and dirty (wet in both cases). A better indication would be a pressure drop as the filter becomes clogged. This is accomplished by placing pressure

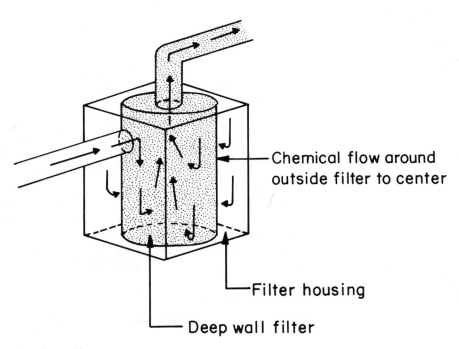

Chemical flow around
outside filter to center

Filter housing

Deep wall filter

Fig. 6-9.   Developer filter.

gauges before and after the filter. Differential pressure gauges are also available.

In-depth filters are made of pressed cellulose or natural fibers. There is also a cord or rope style. In all cases, if a filter is rated at 25 μm, it will stop a 25-μm particle (or larger) regardless of design. (As the scale gets smaller, the price increases.) Often the cord type with its cross-lacing is thought to be less efficient because of its obvious large holes. The primary filtering is in the cord itself. Pore size is rated in micrometers (μm) but is commonly referred to as microns (μ). The smallest particle the human eye can see, unaided, is 40 μ. Water is filtered at the treatment plant to about 90 μm; water to mixing valves must be filtered to 5 to 10 μm to protect the thermostatic motor mechanism.

The function of a filter is to remove debris that could cause a problem. The developer is often filtered so that gelatin will not coat the temperature control components and transport rollers. Gelatin in the developer tank can be from 50 to 150 μm. To remove algae would require a 1 μm or smaller filter, which is not recommended. There are other, more effective ways to combat algae, as discussed previously. Replenishment and water filters protect their respective mechanisms. The dryer filter, if present, is used to keep dust from being blown onto the damp, sticky film. The primary problem is caking when too small a pore size is used or too much debris accumulates on the outer surface of a filter. This blocks all flow and can lead to sensitometric problems and even mechanical problems such as a burned-out pump.

Replenishment/Regeneration System

Function

The replenishment/regeneration system replenishes the chemical volume to keep the tanks full. Chemicals are carried out in the film emulsion layers. Water is evaporated out during prolonged use without feeding films (standby). Should the volume be lowered, the immersion time will change and roller squeegee efficiency could be affected. The results would be a change in sensitometry and/or transport problems including stain, spotting, run down, and run back. This system also serves to regenerate the chemical activity that is being depleted as the film passes through the chemical stages. Development means the oxidation of the developer so that the released electrons can reduce the exposed silver halide crystals to metallic silver and thus convert the latent image into the visible image. The developer is also depleted by long hours of heating and agitation (standby). The fixer accumulates developer, brought in by the film, and silver cleared out of the emulsion. The wash water accumulates fixer. Regeneration is the process in which these chemicals are replaced in order to sustain a certain activity level.

Design

Replenishment (and regeneration) are based on the square centimeters (square inches) of film density. A mechanism is used to sense the presence of film and activate a pump. The sensor is usually a mechanical switch. Light switches are just now being used in x-ray, although they have been used in other areas of photography for about 10 years.

The sensor responds to the presence of a film by activating a pump that draws chemicals from a storage or replenishment tank. The chemicals are pumped into the processor. As long as film is tripping or activating the sensor, the pump runs. This constitutes a direct metering approach.

A time-based system is also called a proportional or percentage system, accumulation, or modified batch system. The sensor activates a timer that runs (instead of the pump). After a period of film-feeding time (usually based on a length of film), the timer is programmed to activate the pump.

Direct metering is based primarily on film length and does not allow for width or density. The timer-based system introduced in the late 1960s by Hope (Profexray processors) have gained almost universal acceptance today. The timer replenishes a larger quantity of chemicals after a variety of films (widths and density) have been processed. Although the time is still based on film length, the replenishment for a large variety should help compensate for the variation of widths and density.

Another variation on a timer-based system is the use of a timer without a film sensor. A timer activates the pump on a time schedule regardless of the amount of film being processed. This is most usually used (and needed) in low-volume processing situations when there is prolonged standby. Thus it is called standby replenishment.

Components

Film sensors are usually, and historically, snap-action microswitches that require only a "micro" distance (usually 0.001 inches) before they are open or closed. They may be very small or very large overall. Magnetic reed switches require a magnet to be moved passed a glass envelope. Inside are two strips of metal in close proximity but not touching. When a film is fed, the magnet is moved toward the strips, pulling them together and allowing electricity to pass to the replenishment pump. Hope processors pioneered an air switch. When the airflow was broken by a film, a diaphragm would fall, allowing a microswitch to turn on. Light-emitting diode (LED) array connected to a photocell works when the light to the cell is blocked by the presence of film and the timer or pump is activated.

In earlier processors, the microswitch (a single one for replenishment and two to sense double films) was centered over the entrance-to-developer crossover. In this location, it often malfunctioned because chemical debris tended to freeze it and keep it from moving. With time, processor manufacturers moved the switch from the center position to the outside and used two. If one failed, the other would still work. Next came various attempts to place the switch so that chemical fumes and splashes would not reach the switch.

Pumps are of three different types: diaphragm, centrifugal, and bellows. From the early 1960s to mid-1970s, the common pump was the Gorman-Rupp two-solution diaphragm metering pump. This pump was composed of two diaphragm pump heads that moved up or down in relation to a fluted umbrella cam. As the cam rotated, it would alternately press and release the diaphragm, causing the pumping action. Poppet valves let chemicals flow in and out. If the diaphram was next to a narrow part of the cam flute (raised up), it pumped a lower volume; if the pump head was by the wider part of the flute, a larger quantity would be pumped. These pumps originally had a maximum capacity of 80ml/minute but were increased to 200 and finally 800ml/minute. The size increased as processors were speeded up. Faster cycles do not necessarily require more chemicals, but replenishment must take place in a shorter period of time because of the more rapid transport of the film through the detector switch (film sensor). These diaphragm pumps are very susceptible to head pressure variation, which is the change in pressure associated with the height of the solution in the replenishment tank (Fig. 6-10). When the tank is full, more chemicals are pumped per film than when the tank is empty. For this reason, the pump setting is always made when the replenishment tank is half full. Then, from full to empty, an averaging takes place. This remedy only works in a very large department that fills and consume the bulk of the replenisher chemicals daily.

As these pumps wear out, they should be discarded and replaced by the Gorman-Rupp bellows pump, which is made by the same company. The bellows pump is less expensive, will last longer, and is virtually unaffected by the head pressure variation. The diaphram pump used in some Profexray-Litton processors was activated by a timer, ran at high capacity, and by design was not head pressure sensitive. Centrifugal magnetic-drive pumps are not metering pumps and thus are inefficient.

Timers range from 1 to 10 minutes in length of a cycle. If a 10-minute timer operates a pump for 4 minutes in every 10-minute period of film-feeding time, it is operating the pump 40% of the film-feeding time. These timers are usually adjustable.

Replenishment tanks must be calibrated and rechecked monthly. Calibration means filling the tank from empty to full using a graduated bucket or other vessel. As the tank is filled, it will distort, causing the dimensions to change. Molded or stenciled markings are placed on the tanks based on

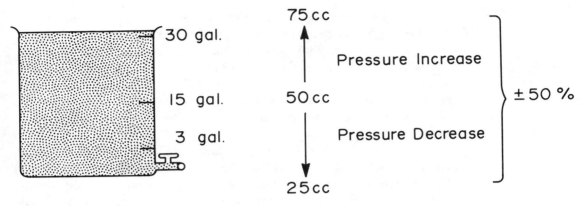

Fig. 6-10.   Head pressure fluctuation.

a mathematical formula and do not allow for the weight of the chemicals, which is about 1 kg/L, (8 pounds/gallon). Tanks generally are cylindrical, as supplied with the processor. However, various sizes and shapes are available to meet specific needs. Replenishment tanks must have floating lids or min-ifloats (hollow balls) to control developer oxidation and fixer fume production. The further away a tank is placed from the processor, the less influence head pressure variation has on the pump efficiency. If one tank supplies two or more processors, it is advisable to install separate bulkhead fittings and lines rather than to run one line with a T. To prevent debris such as hair, paper, etc. from entering the replenishment line and clogging the poppet valves, pump head, and/or flow meters, an in-line filter is used. This filter is a fine metal mesh. Clean it monthly.

Poppet valves are rubber, arrow-shaped devices mounted in a plastic nose cone. The pointed part of the valve points from where the chemicals are coming from. When the pump draws, the poppet base is pulled away from its seal and chemicals are drawn into the pump body. At the same time, the exit poppet is held shut by gravity. On the push cycle, the inlet poppet is sealed and the exit poppet pushed out of the way. Poppet valve material is primarily made of Hypalon made by E.I. du Pont de Nemours & Company. It is impervious to most chemicals but does deteriorate in acetic acid, as found in the fixer. Gorman-Rupp now offers about six different poppet materials to meet specific needs. These are color coded, but the black valve made of ethylenepropylenetriamine (EPT) seems to hold up very well in photographic chemicals.

Establishing Rates

Replenishment and regeneration are based on the square centimeters (inches) of film density processed. Larger film and/or greater density level would require a rate increase. However, the amount of time the developer is heated and agitated (standby) affects the developer strength, so that regeneration is added to try to compensate. A general rule might be 60 to 65ml/14 inches (14 × 17) for 300 films (14 × 17 or equivalent) processed in 8 to 10 hours (with subsequent shutdown). Should the running time become longer (12, 16, or 24 hours), then the replenishment rate would be raised to fight aerial oxidation and evaporation. If the number of films becomes less, the rate would be raised. If exposure tube collimation is used strictly, there will be less image and density on the film, allowing a lower rate to be used.

Developer is critical to the quality of the visible-image radiograph. It must not be either too strong or too weak. The replenishment/regeneration system must be adjusted so that the tank stays full and the activity is held constant. The developer costs about 5 to 10% of the price of film (not including the expense of workers to form a latent image), so good quality and sufficient quantity are not cost restrictive. Assuming little aerial oxidation due to many hours on standby, the primary judgment of adequate developer regeneration is the level of bromide ions. Stable developer should contain about 6 g/L of bromide ions. A level above 8 g/L is due to underreplenishment; a level closer to 4 g/L is due to overreplenishment. During underreplenishment, the developer becomes weaker and will age faster, with a result of a loss in shoulder (H&D) density and contrast. Overreplenishment will tend to drive the curve to the right, producing chemical fog and clumping, which looks like quantum mottle. Bromide determinations may be performed in the institution's laboratory or by the film or chemical manufacturer. The only way to detect aerial oxidation due to prolonged periods of standby in the clinical sense is through careful sensitometric quality control monitoring. The hydroquinone can be measured in the laboratory, but the procedure is quite lengthy and is best performed by a manufacturer. Developer replenishment rates range from 45 to 100ml/14 inches (14 × 17), with 60ml being a starting point. Fixer replenishment is measured by the amount of silver held in balance. Normal stability is achieved in 4 to 6 g/L (about 0.4 to 0.6 troy ounces/gallon). Silver may be measured using silver estimating paper.

A silver level of 2 to 4 g/L indicates overreplenishment and is a sign of waste of fixer. A silver level over 8 g/L indicates underreplenishment, which will lead to film quality problems. Normal replenishment rates per 14 inches (14 × 17) are 85 to 110ml, with 90ml being a starting point. Higher volume per unit of time will allow a lower rate. Fixer replenishment rates have no relationship to the developer replenishment rate. In manual processing, the guideline is a fixer rate that is twice the developer rate. Should that happen in a modern processor, it is a coincidence.

The wash water is not replenished via a pump, so it is usually not considered a part of the replenishment/regeneration system. However, the water must be replenished and refreshed so that it can perform its chemical function of flushing out the residual chemicals, most notably the fixer, to protect the film in long-term storage (archival quality). Water should flow at about 3.5 to 7.5 L/minute (1 to 2 gallons/minute). This volume is not necessary to dilute the 2 to 5% of the fixer carried into the wash tank but to provide sufficient agitation to aid the dilution process. Where water must be conserved, a water recirculation pump and system may be added for $100 to $200. This provides the agitation so the replenishment volume can be lowered to about 2 L/minute (0.5 gallons/minute).

Setting and Measuring Rates

Rates should be set and measured when replenishment tanks are half full so that the average point of head pressure variation is chosen. This is critical for diaphragm and centrifugal pumps. Bellows pumps are generally head pressure insensitive, so it is not important. Rates should only be set or adjusted by the processing specialist or quality control technologist. The level of solution in the replenishment tank should be recorded. Some pumps tend to be inaccurate, and some tend to be nonreproducible. Thus, it is always useful to note the rate set or measured versus the volume of replenisher in the replenishment tank.

Rate Variation

Head pressure variation is the major cause of inaccurate and nonreproducible replenishment rates. When a replenishment tank is full, such as 114 L (30 gallons) in a 115-L tank, the solution level is about 91 cm (36 inches) above the floor, approximately the height of the solution level inside the processor. Thus if the replenishment pump were activated, it would have a column of replenisher fluid pushing down on one side (inlet) and an equal column of working fluid pushing down on the other (outlet) side. The pump would perceive no difference and would deliver its quantity of solution. Columns of fluid are discussed, since volume is not important. As the replenisher chemicals are used, the volume in the replenisher tank falls and the pressure becomes less and less. But the pressure in the processor remains constant or static. Thus the pump no longer has a balance of pressures and delivers less and less chemical for a given setting. This is the significance of head pressure variation.

When selecting a rate, take into consideration the size of the replenishment tank, its location, and the frequency at which it is refilled. A larger tank can produce greater head pressure variation unless it is located 3 m (10 feet) or more away or if the tank is kept full. In photoprocessing, the rule is to mix a small quantity (of replenisher chemicals) frequently. In a 114-L (30-gallon) tank, if about 19 to 38 L (5 to 10 gallons) are added daily to the tank then the head pressure variation is minimized. If the 114-L (30-gallon) tank never falls below 60 L, then this becomes the lowest pressure level. Halfway between 60 and 114 L, or about 90 L, becomes the center point between high and low pressure for setting the replenishment rate.

Pumps fail because of age or dirt. Usually they simply fatigue. Remember that any pump is composed of a pump head, coupler, and an electric motor. Do not discard the entire pump if the pump head has failed, since this usually is the least expensive component. Sometimes excessive heat will warp pump bodies, allowing leaks. If an air leak develops on the inlet side of the pump, the pump will draw in air, reducing the volume of replenisher and causing oxidation in the developer. If the leak occurs on the pump outlet side, chemicals will leak or spray out. This pressure drop means that less chemical will reach the processor tanks. In many pumps, the poppet valves are a part of the pump. The poppet tip can break off, allowing the valve to leave its holder or to jam. Poppets should be inspected quarterly and replaced annually. Inspect to make certain that there are no line kinks or clogs. Clean the replenishment line filter monthly.

Detector-sensor switches located over the developer area will accumulate chemical debris. Keep these clean using a toothbrush. Work them manually up and down each morning to make sure they are free. These units cannot be lubricated except by reducing friction through cleaning and breaking up crystals. Wire trip switches must be checked for bends, twists, or distortion. Finger-type switches like those found on the entrance detector assembly of Kodak X-OMAT M6-AN, M6-A, and M7 must be inspected for alignment and freedom of movement. LEDs may need to be cleaned of dust or moisture so their light reaches the pickup head. In most cases, these switches seldom fail electrically but frequently fail mechanically, resulting in over- or underreplenishment.

Direct metering, as noted above, is the more common method of replenishment by which every film fed into the processor activates the pump, via the sensor switch, and a quantity of chemicals is pumped into the processor. In a timer-based system, the film being fed activates a clock that accumulates film-feeding time (this is a critical phase). At a calculated and preset point, the timer activates the pump. In direct metering, the pump must start and stop. Replenishment is only a function of film length. Thus, for a piece of film of a certain density there may result over- or underreplenishment. Timer-based systems turn on the pump less frequently, tending to minimize mechanical error. The larger quantity of chemical is an average of the film being processed. Timer-based systems should produce a more stable chemical, but they may cause gross underreplenishment in a low-volume situation unless adjusted properly.

Centralized replenishment is usually tied to centralized mixing, although premix could be provided by a dealer. From a tank, lines are run to various processors. Because of the location and size of the central tank, head pressure variation is usually eliminated, thus improving pumping accuracy. In one design, the pumps might be eliminated and replaced with high-quality flow meters. Centralized chemical mixing and distribution save floor space, reduce clutter, and remove a hazard and service problem (replenishment tanks) from the light-room area around a processor. Centralized systems may be installed in new or older institutions but obviously would be less expensive if incorporated in new construction. Centralized silver recovery and chemicals recovery should also be considered. Finally, these systems are expensive but economically justifiable based on consistent quality, floor space, and personnel use. Design service is available from the Seneca Company in Rochester, NY, and the Du Pont Company, Wilmington, DE. Du Pont has a brochure on centralized chemical mixing distribution and recovery written by the author of this book.

Dryer System

Function

The function of the dryer system is to dry out the film by removing the water from the surface and from inside the film. This is accomplished by blowing warm, dry air at the film (Fig. 6-11). In addition, the rollers of the transport system act, in the reverse of the printing concept, to pick up moisture and cast it off to the surrounding dry air. The dryer should function at the least level of heat consistent with dry films. Overdrying will damage the film and can alter the sensitometric values.

Components

The blower is also called a squirrel cage. It is made of a drum with many vanes. With time, the vanes will become coated with dust or chemicals, resulting in less air volume and velocity. The drum is driven at several hundred revolutions per minute by a motor. The drive connection may be direct or

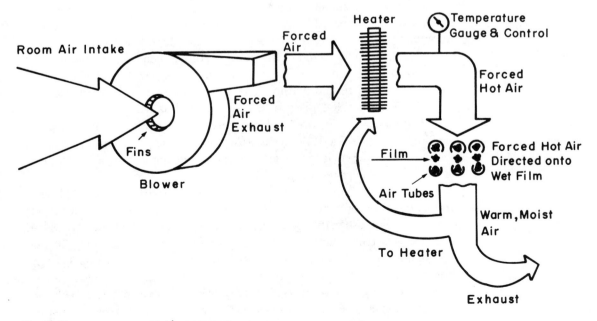

Fig. 6-11.   Air/dryer system.

indirect by belts and sheaves (often called pulleys). Alignment of the belt should be checked when the unit is running. Tension should be snug but never as tight as possible. Tension of belts is usually achieved by moving the motor away from the blower.

Air is moved over a heater and into an air-distribution chamber often called an air plenum. The plenum distributes air to the air tubes, if included. The air tubes either have inserts to ensure that the air velocity is equal across the length of the tube (width of the dryer chamber) or that the air is delivered from both sides. In either case, the air velocity does not blow moisture off the film but keeps the air moving away from the film as it picks up moisture.

Heaters are rated in watts (volts × amperes), and there usually are two to three units of 1550 to 2500 W. In general, heaters draw about 10 A and constitute the single major (60 to 80%) user of electricity. Heaters are usually wired on 220-V lines, except in smaller tabletop units. The heaters get very hot as air is blown across them. Thus, to achieve 55°C (130°F) in the dryer chamber, the heater must be 95 to 125°C (203 to 257°F). A safety thermostat rated at 121°C (250°F) is located directly over the heaters. If the air or control thermostat fails, the safety thermostat opens the heater circuit to prevent damage or fire.

The safety thermostat is generally an automatic reset unit and should seldom ever "blow." The higher the setting, the longer the cool-down and recycle period. These units are generally a bimetallic snap disk. The control thermostat is usually activated by the expansion or contraction of a gas, such as ether, in a sensing probe. As the temperature rises, the gas expands and opens the switch (see the temperature control system section above). When the safety thermostat fails, the control thermostat will appear broken.

Rollers are a part of the transport system, and yet they contribute to drying. Dryer rollers are almost always a porous material such as phenolic or sponge. This is important because they act like wipers, picking up moisture and passing it into the surrounding dry air, which accepts the moisture. The circumference of 2.54-cm (1.0 inch) diameter rollers is 8 cm (3.14 inch), based on the following formula: circumference = pi × diameter. Pi is the mathematical constant 3.14. The surface area for one 17-inch-long roller 1 inch in diameter is 136 cm² (53.4 inch²).

Factors Affecting Efficiency

Air intake quality will vary from one institution to another, one area to another within a hospital, and throughout the day and year. Quality refers to the ambient air temperature, moisture, and dirt. If the air is cool and moist (high relative humidity), it must be warmed up and dried out, a less efficient system than natural conditions of warm (70°F) and dry (40%RH) air. Dirty air is inefficient because the dirt (dust) can plate on the blower blades and coat and insulate heaters and the thermostat. The dirt reduces airflow and can block air tubes.

Air heating is the function of the heater element, which produces about 2000 to 3000 W of power and about 122°C (250°F). If two or three heaters are used, make certain all units are working. If one is broken, the processor will feel warm but will not efficiently dry films.

The air to be heated, the heated air circulation, and the exhaust all are functions of the blower. Blowers typically move about 5.7 m³/minute (200 cfm). Should the drive belt break, the blower will not move air and the element will overheat, turning off the control thermostat and/or the safety thermostat. When the blower fins get dirty, the cage can get out of balance and destroy the drive belt, blower bearings, and/or motor bearings. If the blower is inefficient or at least cannot overcome exhaust tube resistance, then moisture will back up in the dryer, causing wet films. If the exhaust is drawing air in excess of the blower rating, the blower motor and heater can be damaged. Airflow is measured with a velometer.

Exhaust is usually at the bottom of the air plenum and the processor because warm air rises. However, the exhaust air might be about 40°C (100°F), in which case it would be reluctant to be pushed toward the exhaust. Also, as it exits, it cools rapidly and its velocity drops. It has been estimated that for every bend in air exhaust duct there is a 15 to 50% loss in air velocity. Distance and temperature differentials also reduce velocity. To overcome these inefficiencies, exhaust duct with a 10-cm (4-inch) diameter should be used. The run should have the fewest number of bends, and the bends should be gentle (100°, 120° rather than 90°). Dust can collect in the exhaust duct. If the processor (internal) exhaust duct becomes disconnected, inefficiency can result. Some older units have dampers, which should be partially open at the top to create a natural heat rise. If the dampers are too open, are set in the wrong direction, or are closed, drying problems will result.

Wet Film Problems

Electromechanically, wet films will be produced if the heat or blower is not functioning. This may be due to a faulty control or safety thermostat, heater, blower, blower motor (the motor often has its own circuit breaker), or thermometer. Mechanically, if the rollers are dirty (glazed with gelatin) then moisture pickup will be reduced. If rollers are not properly installed or if drive gears are of the wrong diameter, film will fall rapidly through vertical dryer chambers and emerge damp. In all of these cases, the film will be soft and cool and will take several minutes to dry or require a second passage through the dryer.

When the exhaust is blocked or inefficient, the type of wet film is unique. The film is hard and generally warm, and the moisture sits on the surface of the film. Wave the film in room air, and the moisture disappears in about 15 seconds. The moisture in this case is atomized mist. Moisture removed from previous films (an important clue) builds up in the dryer instead of being exhausted. Finally a hard (chemically) and dry (dryer) film passes through this cloud of moisture near the bottom of the dryer chamber, and the moisture clings to the dry film. Out of the processor, the moisture leaves the film and moves into the drier room air. Refer to the note above about an important clue: This phenomenon usually occurs after running many films or all large-format films such as serial exams. As the moisture builds up, the trailing edge will become damp, then the next film will exhibit the last quarter wet, etc. When exhaust problems are suspected, disconnect the exhaust duct in the darkroom, allowing easier exit of the exhaust air and moisture. If this works, then install a larger-diameter exhaust duct, reduce the number of bends or the sharpness of bends, and/or consider installing a small fan to help draw out the exhaust air. If an air break has been installed, reduce the size of the opening or eliminate it.

Chemical-induced wetness is like the electromechanical wetness: The gelatin is soft, cool, and soggy and takes a long time to dry. The developer hardener is usually the primary suspect as the cause of wet films and not the fixer hardener. To ascertain if the fixer could be the cause, perform a clearing time test in the fixer. If this appears normal, discard the developer and refill with fresh.

Temperature is really an electromechanical component but has special influence on wet films. If the developer temperature is over 35°C (95°F), the emulsion can swell to a greater thickness than the hardeners can control. Very few processors have an active or positive fixer temperature control, so the fixer temperature drifts throughout the day from room temperature at start-up to as high as 40°C (104°F) by early evening. As the fixer temperature approaches the higher temperature, the hardeners cannot control the swelling and wet films result. Thus it is important to monitor fixer temperature periodically at the end of a workday or when wet films show up only at the end of the day. There are ways to control the higher fixer temperature problems, such as tank insulation and/or the addition of a heat exchanger.

Electrical System

Function

This system provides the power to the other five electromechanical systems that support the chemistry system. It is composed of conductors and switches that move the electricity around and consumers such as motors, heaters, and lamps. Most processors consume 4 to 5 kW/hour and operate on 120/240 VAC and 15 to 25 A.

Working with Electricians

The purpose of this section is not to help someone to be an electrician or to do electrical repairs, but rather to help a technologist in discussing problems with the electrician or repair person. The electrician is often at a disadvantage because he or she understands electrical systems but not the x-ray processor or what the various functions are. In this latter case, the electrician is a layperson. The repair person might be inclined to replace an electrical component without the knowledge or interest to investigate why it failed electrically. In both cases, there is potential for lost efficiency and economy. It is very advantageous if the processing specialist or quality control technologist can discuss electrical problems with the electrician. For instance, if a pump fails, would the electrician be allowed to replace the complete $400 assembly or be asked to test the motor, connectors, plugs, etc. to see if the motor is okay? The motor is the most expensive part. It would be an unnecessary expense to replace the whole pump or even the motor if the problem were simply a shorted-out plug caused by some moisture getting inside. The electrician could repair the plug in 15 minutes. What if only the starting condenser were bad or the starting relay? These are $15 items replaced in minutes. What if only the starting windings were bad or the wrong fuse was used. Should the processor be shut down or should options be discussed with the electrician? Most often, temporary repairs, bypasses, etc. can be safely worked by the electrician.

Safety

Continuing with the theme above, it is very hazardous and counterproductive simply to replace broken electrical components without trying to find out why they failed and, if necessary, make changes to prevent future failure. The classic example is the replacement of fuses. Fuses are safety devices. When there is an abnormally high current, the fuse "burns up" before the motor or heater does, thus saving the more expensive component.

When working on any electrical component, be sure the power is off. Turn off the processor. Next go to the main isolator (circuit breaker, fuse box, power supply) and open the circuit. Next put a lock on the box or terminal and a tag or sign to tell another person that the switch must be left open. Then test to make sure the switch is really locked out. Next test the processor to see if it will turn on. Then remove the cover of the electrical panel and test with an instrument for the presence of electricity. This is the standard "lock, tag, test" procedure.

Always try to work with a partner. If there is any chance of a shock, rethink the work procedure to eliminate the potential. If live electricity is being monitored with a meter, make certain that, should there be a chance for an electrical shock, the electricity does not enter the right side of the body and exit on the left side (or vice versa), passing through the heart. Make certain that clothes and shoes are dry. Stand on a thick rubber, plastic, or wooden platform to insulate. These are aspects of the "keep your left hand in your pocket" safety rule to prevent electricity from passing through the heart. Contrary to popular belief, very small amounts of current can kill.

Components

Switches open and close (also called "make and break"). They can be manually or automatically activated. A normally open (NO) switch is one found not to pass electricity when electricity is applied. Someone must close the switch or some other sequence must precede the closing. When the processor is turned on, the switch is closed and electricity passes to other stages or areas or circuits. One circuit would be replenishment. The switch has both an NO and a normally closed (NC) circuit. When a film is fed, the NO circuit is closed, turning on the replenishment pump and opening the NC circuit, resetting the time-delay timer. After the film passes the switch, the switch returns to its normal position, opening the NO, which turns off the pump and recloses the NC, which starts the timer for the time delay. The time delay may be a motor or a relay, but at the end of, typically, 3 seconds, it closes another NO switch, which passes electricity to another NO switch called a bell. On-off switches are referred to as rocker switches because the switch (activator) rocks back and forth (as opposed to toggle or lever or push button). It is also called a throw switch because one "throws" it to the on or off position (as opposed to movement or slide switches). They have one circuit or two circuits referred to as poles. Each circuit or pole has two posts: electricity to the switch and electricity out of the switch. Thus, the normal terminology would be single-throw single-pole (STSP) or single-throw double-pole (STDP) switch. A double-pole switch carries two separate circuits, which can be of different voltages.

Conductors or wires are coated with insulation that can fail with heat and time. Where the wires connect to terminals, corrosion can block electrical passage or terminals can become loose. Conductors are usually color coded and/or numbered. Some processors have labels on power cords. In the United States, black (K) indicates primary hot wires, red (R) would be secondary hot, white (W) is neutral, and green (G) is safety ground. Most processors sold in Canada are made in the United States. Internationally, the electrical code is brown (BRN) for primary, purple (P) for secondary, and green with a yellow strip (G-Y) for safety ground. Neutral, where used, must not be connected to ground except in the lock-out box.

Consumers of electricity include heaters, motors, and lamps. Consumption is in kilowatts of power per hour. A watt is derived by multiplying the voltage times the amperage. Dryer heaters run from 1000 to 7500 W and account for 75% of the processor consumption. Developer heaters run from 500 to 2000 W. Motors draw about 0.08 to 0.2 kW/hour.

Schematic

An electrical schematic shows the general layout of the components and sequence in a stylized grid (Fig. 6-12). It tells what is on which circuit or switch. It easily allows one to determine voltage requirements to a motor. It

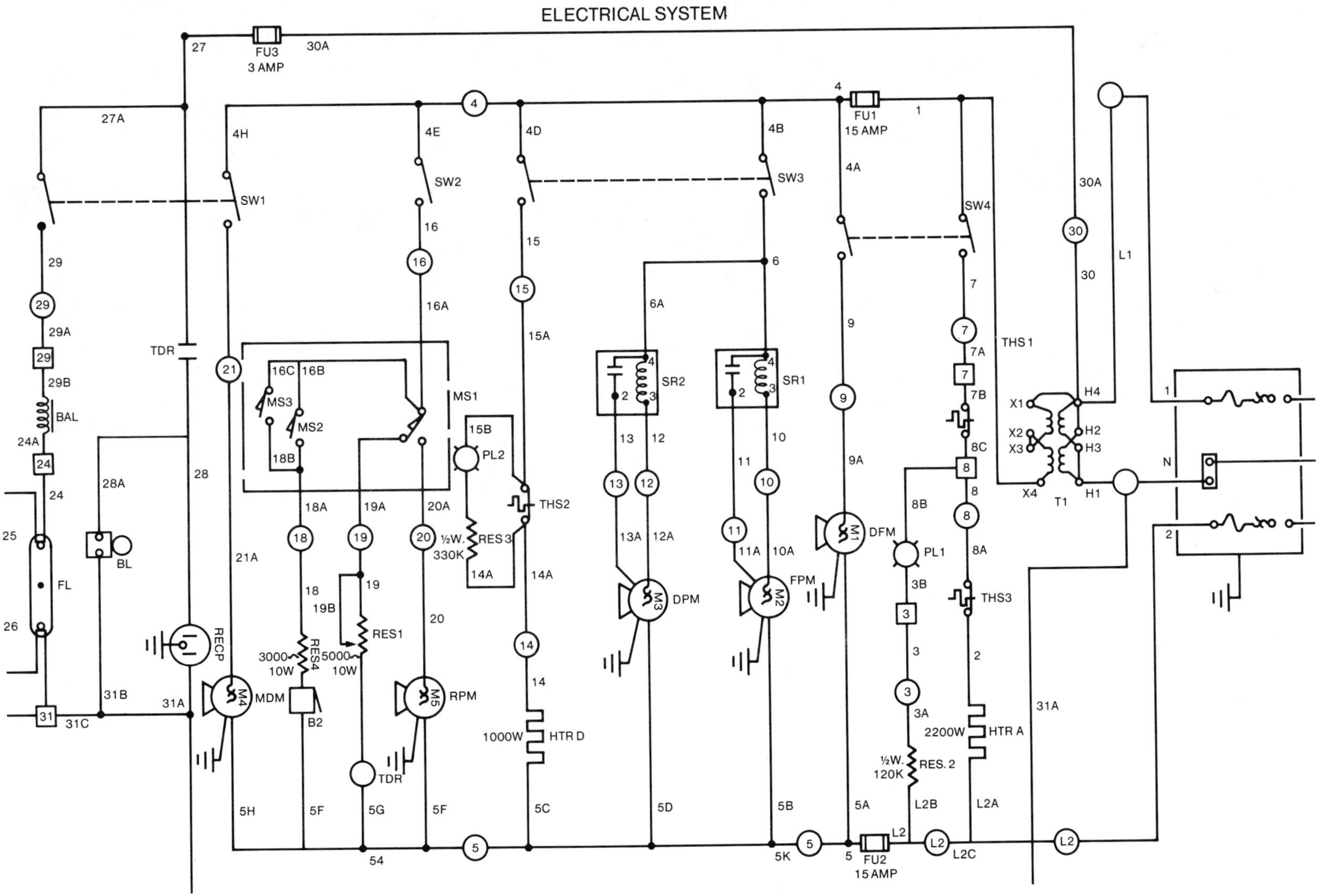

Fig. 6-12. Electrical system.

aids in troubleshooting by guiding one through the steps and sequences of operation. There is no scale or relative position of the parts.

Wiring Diagrams

Wiring diagrams show the position of wires and devices. They will show the microswitches for replenishment at the top of the page, since these switches are the highest electrical devices inside the processor. If the time-delay bell is located to the left and lower than the main drive motor in the processor, the diagram will reflect this. This is like having "x-ray vision" of the electrical parts. Wires will be numbered and color coded. The only thing not identified is the length of the wire used on a circuit, but that is a minor problem and the diagram will give some hints anyway.

Sometimes the schematic and diagram are combined, either aiding or confusing the worker. In any case, working with the electrical drawings in the processor manual will help the troubleshooter and the student to understand better how, why, and when things work and/or fail. It is often more meaningful to "read" the electrical drawings than to read descriptive words in the processor manual.

Watts of Power

Electricity is sold and used based on kilowatt hours or kilowatts per hour (kW/hour). It is calculated by multiplying volts times amperage. For instance, a developer heater on a 115-VAC circuit drawing 4.35 A would be rated at 500 W or 0.5 kW. Another developer heater wired to a 220-VAC supply line and drawing only 2.3 A would also be a 500-W heater. Usually, developer heaters are wired to 115 VAC and range from 500 to 750 or 1000 W. Some older processors used two 1000-W heaters. Since the heaters are made with standard fittings, they can be interchanged or upgraded as long as the physical size is compatible.

Dryer heaters are usually on a 200-VAC (208, 220, 230) supply and range from one 1000-W heater to three 2500-W heaters. Usually, there are two 1550-W heaters in the X-OMAT M6-AN or M6-AW, or one 2500-W, much as in the older M4. By operating on 200 VAC, less current is needed to produce the same power. When there is more than one heater, one can burn out and the reduced efficiency will produce a damp film, although the dryer might feel sufficiently warm.

Testing

Hot testing means using a test light while the power is turned on to see if electricity is in various circuits or at various terminals. A volt-ohm-milliammeter (VOM) could also be used to detect voltage and to measure the level of the voltage. Care must be exercised to prevent shock.

Cold testing involves testing with all external power turned off and locked out. The VOM is set at ohms, the units of resistance, and a 9-V battery inside the meter is switched on. Touching the meter probes together will send the needle from left to right, from very high to low resistance. When the meter probe is touched to either side of an electrical device, the battery sends electricity through the device (if functional) and a low resistance is measured. If the device is nonfunctional, then it is said to be "open" (goes to ground or another circuit) and there is a very high resistance. Testing the circuit in this way is called continuity checking because the test will indicate a continuous circuit. However, test each part in a circuit separately: Disconnect, pull fuses, or open switches to isolate the one part to be tested.

Chapter 7

Maintenance

Control of Quality

Electromechanical

Use a bimetallic (stem, dial) or electronic (analog or digital) thermometer to monitor the temperature in each of the chemical tanks (developer, fixer, wash) and the dryer. Monitor in the morning and at night. Monitor the transport rate, immersion times, and/or motor or roller revolutions per minute (rpm). Monitor line voltage levels at start-up and when at normal operating levels. Disassemble racks annually to inspect all bearings and shafts for wear. Disassemble all motors and pumps annually to inspect them and repair corrosion. Keep detailed records of findings and repair work. Testing and inspection should be sufficient to indicate potential trouble before it becomes a problem. Frequent testing is important to monitor wear as a part of predictive and preventive maintenance.

Chemical

Developer bromide levels determine if the correct replenishment rate is being used. Hydroquinone determination indicates the amount of aerial oxidation, mixing error, age, etc. but is a difficult test that is best performed by the chemical companies. Specific gravity measures the density of the solution relative to water, which is 1.000 at 23°C (70°F). Specific gravity of developers ranges from 1.070 to 1.100. It is measured using a hydrometer. The density of fixer is 1.077 to 1.110, depending on brand. The pH is a poor indicator of activity or efficiency and is best used as a general indicator of value. A pH meter should be used, preferably one with temperature compensation built in. Be certain to buffer (calibrate) the unit to pH 10 when reading developers and pH 4 when reading fixers. Narrow-range, color-corrected pH paper is of little value. One product that is used like pH paper and that is very useful is silver estimating paper. The silver content of the fixer can be measured with sufficient accuracy to determine if the fixer replenishment rate is accurate. Another easy fixer test is the clearing time test. Wash water is tested by monitoring its flow rate and temperature. A chemical company can perform a hypo-retention test on a sample film to measure the archival quality.

Sensitometric

The function of the chemicals is to convert the latent image into the visible image. Sensitometry is the quantitative measure of the film's response to exposure and development. If a box of test film is selected and set aside for testing only and if a reproducible exposure (sensitometer) is put on the film and then developed, any changes when compared with a master film will be due to processing variations. These variations could be electromechanical and/or chemical. Sensitometric testing measures the sum total of the efficiency of the electromechanical systems (processor) in controlling the chemical system. Sensitometric testing, then, is the single best tool to use to control quality. Indeed, if the quality is acceptable there is no need to check temperature or replenishment rates.

Initiating a Processing Quality Control Program

Radiographic processing is done in an automated processor to achieve consistent quality. The processing system is a chemical process that has specific conditions of time and temperature based on a given chemical activity. The sum result of processing is the quality of the radiograph produced.

Processing quality control is a procedure of monitoring to see if there is consistency and to what extent there is consistency. Before quality can be improved, there must first be the capability for producing consistent quality. This is because the variables of processing must be identified, their degree of fluctuation and cycling patterns noted, and finally limits of acceptability established. Once the uncontrolled variables are identified, the best corrective measure to be taken to control the variable will become more apparent. Sometimes, the variable may have to be compensated for, minimized, or eliminated. In this process of identifying and controlling the various variables, indications are often revealed about the best way to consistently achieve an optimized quality.

Thus, the basic procedure is to select one processor, identify quality, identify and control all of the variables of the processing system, and establish consistency. Next, select a second processor and match it to the first in quality and consistency.

Then add a third processor. Continue until the entire hospital is controlled so that each processor produces a radiograph of consistent quality within acceptable limits. Although the variables in each processor are about the same, they are independent of one another and will deviate differently. It is for this reason that one should not attempt to try to control all processors at the same time immediately. Even matching many processors at one time is difficult because it entails changing some variables, but the wrong variable might be chosen or might be placed in a situation of greater fluctuation.

Preparation of The Processor

- Clean the processor very thoroughly. Flush out all lines, including the replenishment tubing coming from the replenishment tank.
- Using a checklist, inspect all components of the processor. Inspect alignment and points of wear.
- Correct any mechanical problems. Make note of and order new parts when indicated. Record this information.
- Lubricate all necessary points.
- Mix and install chemistry. Make note of chemistry brand, type, order code or other identification, and serial number. Also note the amount of starter solution added to developer.
- Install a new filter (if used in the processor). Note make, type, and size in micrometers.
- Reassemble the processor and turn the unit on.
- While the processor is coming up to operating condition, clean the outside of the processor, especially the feed tray and receiver bin.

Operational Conditions

- When the processor is functioning normally, make note of and record the following specifications. (Begin with current levels of temperature, etc.)

  Developer immersion time: leading edge into developer chemistry until leading edge exits the developer

  Fixer immersion time

  Wash immersion timer

  Dryer time

  Dry-to-dry time (14 × 17)

Entrance feed time

Exit time (14 × 17) (this added to dry-to-dry time provides Drop-to-Drop time)

Calculate rate of inches per minute

Developer temperature using a calibrated bimetallic or electronic thermometer. Calibrate thermometer on processor

Fixer temperature

Wash temperature

Dryer temperature

Replenishment rate (per 14 × 17 fed 17 inches across and with replenishment tank half full of developer/fixer)

Wash water flow rate

Note ambient conditions

- Make sure that the unit is clean, that it is functioning properly, and that temperature and speed are stabilized by feeding six unexposed 14 × 17 films through the processor. Carefully inspect the last film for artifacts.
- Recheck film-feeding rate and developer temperature and record.
- Observe and comment on chemical circulation and blower functions. Also note activity of any indicator lights
- Make sure no person alters any temperatures or rates in the processor.

Quality Control Test

- With the processor at a controlled "known" state (such as is outlined above), test films can be processed.
- In the darkroom, from a preselected box of film as described elsewhere, flash a film, preferably using a sensitometer. Process it immediately. Feed the film with the exposed area crosswise, parallel to the entrance slot. This reduces the effect of bromide drag.
- After processing, recheck developer temperature for stability and record this finding. While the last film is being fed, the entrance time can be monitored and recorded.

Interpretation

- Some routine patient films should be processed and reviewed to see if they truly represent average or normal films in terms of position, density, contrast, and artifacts.
- The next step:

  If the patient films are unacceptable, make corrections and repeat the test procedure.

  If the patient films are acceptable, then the test film becomes the master film and should be so labeled and filed. Make several copies and file them in separate places in case one film is lost. Record patient film identification numbers in case it is ever necessary to retrieve these films for comparison.

- The master control film now represents average or normal films under the known conditions of processing.
- This should be filed with all available information.

Continuous Monitoring for Consistency

- On a regular basis, such as three times daily or during shifts but at least daily, another film should be sensitometrically exposed and processed.
- This test film is compared with the Master control film.
- Next step:

  If the films do not match but are within acceptable limits, make note of this by recording the density shift. If convenient, recheck all specifications such as temperature. Acceptable limits are ± 15%.

  If films do not match and are beyond acceptable limits, expose a second test film to verify the results. Next, a complete check must immediately be made of all processing conditions to identify which variables are out of limits. Suspend processing patient films until the situation is corrected. Control, readjust, or compensate for the offending variable. Record cause-and-effect relationships. Process another test film to verify that acceptable processing has been regained.

- Periodically, such as weekly, all records must be reviewed and updated and trends noted.

Expansion of Program

- Control test films should be processed before and after any major changes in conditions, such as when chemistry is changed or a drive motor or pump motor is replaced.
- Processing should be consistent. The routine processing of a controlled-exposure film will indicate the degree of consistency and will help to identify variables and the extent that they individually are inconsistent. Before a variable can be controlled, it must be identified.
- When consistent quality processing has been achieved in one processor for a period of one or more months, then consideration should be given to ensuring that optimal quality is being provided. Should a different definition of quality be produced, then the master control film must be replaced with a new film to reflect the new specifications of processing.
- When one processor is proved to be producing consistent quality, then work should begin on establishing the consistency of a second pro-

cessor relative to itself and relative to the first processor. If two processing systems can be held consistent, then the third processor should be added. In each case, the master control film is the controlling factor to which all other test film should be matched.

Types of Programs

Preventive Maintenance

As an engineering principle, preventive maintenance suggests a schedule of rebuilding various components. This is a very expensive and time-consuming procedure, but the belief is that if the equipment is constantly being renewed then failure is less likely to occur. The main problem is that parts do not fail on a scheduled basis. Thus, although many maintenance companies (dealers, solution service, agencies, etc.) offer preventive maintenance, what is usually supplied is a cleaning and parts replacement service. Replacing parts after they have failed obviously has not prevented failure. All work must be recorded and reviewed periodically.

Predictive Maintenance

Predictive maintenance requires much more inspection time and awareness so that as many parts as possible are monitored and recorded. At some point, as wear progresses, the service person will be able to predict failure and thus justify replacing the part to prevent untimely failure. Predictive maintenance is much less costly in parts and time than preventive maintenance, and yet it provides an economical and realistic way to make preventive maintenance work. The key is involvement with the equipment so wear can be seen and monitored. Wear will often progress only so far and then will cease or be dramatically reduced, eliminating the need for a new part. Predictive maintenance allows for jury-rigging, compensation, modification, or change in the equipment to reduce wear factors. Keep detailed records. Look for the obvious and less obvious, consistencies and inconsistencies.

Tailor-Made Programs

What does each processor need in the way of cleaning, lubrication, alignment, adjustment, etc.? Each processor is unique in its work load and location within the institution. Two processors of the same make and model most usually will require different maintenance schedules. The processor manuals often fail to point this out. Certainly one unit processing 100 films per day will not have the same wear and get as dirty as a unit that handles 300 or 500 films per day. What works as a cleaning schedule in one hospital may not work in another. Thus it is very important that the processing specialist or quality control technologist (QCT) develop a custom or tailor-made program. To begin, make an outline of all the components to be inspected, cleaned, lubricated, and aligned. Next check off whether these activities should be performed once, twice, or three times daily. List those items that only need to be checked weekly, biweekly, monthly, quarterly, or yearly. Use personal experience, past history, and recommendations from processor manufacturers. Once the program has been drawn up, stick to it strictly. If the schedule cannot be maintained or if some items are found to be a waste of effort, then make changes, but try to work 4 to 6 weeks before making changes. At each step, the program becomes fine-tuned to meet the needs of a specific processor in a specific institution. It will require time to develop, but in the long run it should be very efficient.

Solution Service

The term *solution service* generally refers to a company that prepares chemicals in bulk and delivers this premix to the hospital. As a part of their service, they also might clean and/or repair the processors. Sometimes they also handle silver reclamation services. Dealers and silver service companies might also offer these services to gain other business. In any case, the institution should have a processing specialist or QCT who is sufficiently trained to be able to work with the service personnel. The service contract should reflect the hospital's needs for each processor rather than a general service contract offered by the dealer. For instance, if it is believed that a high-volume processor should be cleaned every 2 weeks, then that should be the basis of the contract. Cleaning once a month is an unfounded habit, unfortunately. The rule is to keep the processor clean. Thus, the outside people perform their work once or twice a month and the in-house specialist takes care of all other times. The result is a team effort. A more specific contract might cost more than a general contract, but processing is the least expensive component in image formation. When the hired service personnel work within an institution, they must follow the institution's safety policies and procedures. A staff member should always supervise all work to monitor compliance with the contract, to be able to discuss problem areas uncovered, and to ensure safety. Service personnel should note the condition of the processor as found and as it is left, with a written report of observations. Communication between the service person and the hospital are important.

Developing a Service Contract/Job Description

The initial step is to detail all the various jobs to be done, their frequency, and the expected quality. Then decide who will do them. An outside service may be contracted if there is insufficient time or personnel. The institution must decide what it wants done, how it is to be done, and how frequently.

If the contracted service exceeds these requirements, then use the service company's guide. The service contract and in-house specialist should compliment and act as a check-and-balance system to each other while maintaining a team effort. Because many institutions will have different jobs, combined jobs, and/or different titles for various jobs, the following are job descriptions for the processing specialist and QCT.

Job Description for the Processing Specialist

I. Responsibilities

Is responsible for all activities relative to the use, operation, maintenance, repair, and quality of products produced by the automatic processors from a technical standpoint rather than administrative.

Works with and reports to the QCT.

Is responsible for daily maintenance and cleaning. This may be supervisory.

Is responsible for obtaining scheduled sensitometric and other data for analysis by the QCT.

Advises (or repairs if authorized) on the need for service.

Works with outside service and personnel.

Maintains all records relative to the processor.

Holds or participates in regular meetings to discuss and inform others regarding processor problems, processing consistency, and trends. This includes teaching and seminars for staff and students.

Works with the QCT to educate staff and students.

If qualified or authorized to repair all or certain components, then is responsible for developing, ordering, and maintaining an orderly and adequate supply of spare parts.

Is responsible for the use of safety goggles and other safety equipment and procedures as might be required at all times when working on the processor or with chemicals in general.

Is responsible for chemical orders, storage, inventory, mixing, and records.

Maintains all applicable parts and service manuals, tools, and brochures.

II. Other areas that might be included

Silver reclamation service and control.

Darkroom inspection service and record keeping.

Safelight inspection service, repair, and records. Cassette and screen inspection, cleaning, repair, and/or replacement and record keeping. This might be a shared job with the x-ray specialist or QCT.

View-box cleaning, inspection (with light meter), repair, and
record keeping.

Safety inspection and supervision of installation of any or some
pieces of auxiliary equipment.

Teaching students and/or staff about photographic chemistry,
electrical schematic reading, processor, and processing.

III. Background requirements and other considerations

Depending on the level of involvement, the requirements will vary
but generally are as follows:

- High-school diploma or better
- Mechanical and electrical capabilities
- Willingness to learn
- Appreciation for the technical importance of the processor
- A history of safe work habits

A senior darkroom technician (or supervisor) or a technologist
interested in technical factors or in training for QCT position is
preferable.

The person can initially begin by working with an outside service
organization but should eventually (6 months) reduce the need
or eliminate this service.

The person should, after 6 months of practical work experience
and demonstrated motivation, be sent to an advanced school on
processing for a weeklong course in chemistry and processors.

After the first year, consideration should be given to having the
person trained in quality control and sensitometry.

The processing specialist is the in-house authority on the
maintenance, repair, and operation of the processors and
processing. This is a technical position rather than administrative
but should be on a level of a supervisor.

Job Description for the X-ray Quality Control Technologist

I. Responsibilities

Is responsible for all phases of quality control from a technical
standpoint rather than administrative.

Identifies parameters needing control and sets limits.

Monitors to see if parameters are within limits.

Notifies the proper administrator of out-of-limits equipment and/or
conditions and/or procedures.

Holds regular meetings to discuss and inform regarding the quality
control program on various levels: administrative, technical, staff,
and paramedical.

Conducts or assists in educational programs on quality control for
staff and students.

Is responsible for or works with the radiation safety officer.

Attends meetings or training programs of a specific nature to gain and maintain expertise in various areas.

Establishes a file on quality control literature.

Establishes, maintains, and reviews records on the progress of quality control program to identify trends.

Is responsible for or works with the general safety supervisor.

II. Areas of quality control

Storage conditions of film, chemicals, isotopes, and general supplies.

Inventory control, record system, ordering sequences, etc.; processing control and processor maintenance programs.

Exposure control, generator/tube maintenance programs, and screen and cassette monitoring.

View-box control, film sorting and filing.

Technique establishment and review.

Documentation for certification.

Personnel development.

III. Other considerations

The QCT should have technical background and motivation. Registered technologist (RT) (American Registry of Radiologic Technologists [ARRT]) certification should be the minimal qualification. B.S. degree would be preferred.

The QCT should be allowed to devote at least 50% of his or her time to a quality control program in a small institution (200 beds or less) and full time in larger institutions. Institutions with more than 500 beds may require part-time or full-time helpers working under the QCT. The time factor is required to allow for sufficient monitoring and tests.

The QCT identifies problems from a technical standpoint. An administrator or supervisor decides on the degree and method of correction of the problem. This is important in the problem of staff motivation and authority chains.

The QCT should be on the same authority level as the chief technologist or administrative assistant depending on job classification within a given institution. In larger institutions, it might be possible, depending on an individual's credentials, to have an administrative director and a technical director.

The QCT should be aware of the regulations of and serve as liaison with all local, state, and national radiation, occupational, and environmental groups (Bureau of Radiologic Health, Occupational Safety and Health Administration [OSHA], Environmental Protection Agency [EPA], Joint Commission on Accreditation of Hospitals [JCAH]).

Maintenance Schedule

Theory

It is vital to patients' health that a radiograph be of the very best diagnostic quality time after time. This consistency of quality is called quality control or quality assurance. The film quality is controlled by the chemicals, which are in turn controlled by the electromechanical devices and systems. Therefore, quality control includes a preventive maintenance program.

When a film is repeated, the patient receives additional radiation and the department suffers financial waste and inefficiency.

In general, technologists work with the patient and exposure equipment to create a latent or hidden image. This image is of no value unless correctly developed into a visible image. Development amplifies the original signal many million times, fixing removes undeveloped crystals, the wash water removes the remaining chemicals, and the dryer removes the water.

All of these steps together constitute processing, and they must be highly controlled. Thus, processing is a chemical reaction that occurs in an electromechanical device, the processor. It is extremely important to remember that it is inadequate just to fix a part. Consideration must be given to how that part, whether fixed or broken, influences the radiograph.

General Considerations

- Safety
  The developer is hazardous.
  Wear safety glasses or goggles at all times.
  Wash your hands frequently.
  Wear rubber gloves, an apron, and safety shoes or boots as needed.
  Make sure the area is well lighted and ventilated, and know the location of an eyewash station.
  Lock out, tag, and test the mains isolator (electrical control box).
  Secure the work area against onlookers.
  Plan the work.
  Be mindful of pinch points and loose clothing.

Daily

- At start-up
  Remove crossovers and guide shoes (deflector plates) and wash them in warm water with a sponge or plastic cleaning pad.[1]*
  Wash all rollers attached to deep racks that are out of solution to remove dirt, gelatin, debris, and crystals.

  * Notes begin on p. 136.

Clean all interior surfaces.

Check the processor tank solution level. Top off (fill) if low. If persistent, determine the cause and correct it. Record quantity added.

Check replenishment tank levels, color, odor, and lines to processors.

Turn the unit on. If it is equipped with multiple switches, turn on the loudest system (dryer) last to allow for inspection of each system (look for agitation, check replenishment and time delay relay, and check transport). Turn on the water next to last and observe the tank filling or time it. Correct any problems. Install crossovers and guides.

Clean and install all fume control hoods and splash guards, and close the lid.

Feed four 35 × 43-cm (14 × 17-inch), green, unprocessed films to clean up rollers. Do not use preprocessed black films, because they are harder and contain fixer.

Clean exterior surfaces including the feed tray and receiver bin.

Wash off all darkroom work surfaces.

When the unit achieves operating conditions, feed a 20 × 25-cm (8 × 10-inch) sensitometrically exposed film.[2] Record the processing conditions. Compare the processed test film to the master film (standard). Record and correct artifact and image quality problems.

Save the film as a record. If correction is required, process another test film and recheck.

- During work period

Operators should be trained to be aware of normal processor aspects such as vibration, noise level and type, heat, smell, moisture, odors, film-feeding characteristics (speed, angle, pull, etc.), time-delay signal, etc. Any abnormal change should be reported.

If no films are to be processed for a period of 2 hours or longer, the unit should be turned off, including the main power and water. This is ecologically sound and also prolongs the life of the chemistry and processor. Open the lid and remove the fume control hood. Do this even if the unit is equipped with standby (manual or automatic) and/or water- or energy-saving devices.

After any period of 30 minutes or longer in which no films have been fed, a cleanup[3] film should be fed and inspected prior to feeding patient films.

Staff members should not lean against or on the unit.

Films must not be removed unless they have dropped into the receiver bin.

Wipe off the feed tray and receiver bin at midday (or more frequently).

Feed a quality control test film at midday. Correct if needed. Record information.

- At Shutdown

Observe and note the heat level, noise level, vibration, solution levels, replenishment tank level, agitation, cleanliness, transport system, tubing, leaks, etc. prior to turning the unit off. Record problems for correction before next start-up.

Run a quality control test film. Record.

Turn the unit off, starting with the loudest component (water,[4] dryer, transport, etc.).

Remove, inspect, and clean the fume control hood, baffles, splash guards, crossovers, and guide shoes (deflector plates) as at start-up.

Wash all rollers out of solution.

Wash off all chemical splatters[5] and all interior surfaces.

Inspect, wash, or clean chemical debris from the main drive shaft or drive mechanism gears. Relubricate if needed but avoid excess.

Place all removed components in a cabinet or on a shelf protected by a dustcover. If put back into the processor, they will become dirty from fumes and condensation.

Leave the top lid open at least 1 inch at the dryer end by lifting and moving it toward the feed end. Do not lift and rotate the lid, as this leaves a point sticking out.

Wipe down all exterior surfaces.

Restock film, chemicals, and other supplies as required. Record all work.

Weekly

Check the developer, water (on the mixing valve), and dryer thermostats and thermometers for accuracy and response against a known (calibrated) thermometer.[6] Calibrate by removing the front cover (most units) of thermometers or by repositioning the knob or markings on thermostats. Record.

Check the replenishment pump setting, rates, accuracy, and reproducibility against the quantity of chemicals in the replenishment tank. Replenishment pumps are sensitive to head pressure variations and are influenced by quantity, distance, type of tank, etc.[7]

Perform daily shutdown. Remove the developer rack (use proper safety precautions and control drips). Wash it under warm water using a sponge, brush (nonmetallic), or plastic cleaning pad (do not use on soft rollers). When it is clean, rinse it with hot water and inspect each roller, the drive mechanism, turnaround assembly, guide shoes, rack squareness, and tie bar tightness. Make corrections or adjustments as needed. Rinse the rack with hot water and return it to the processor. Record all work and observations.

Lubricate the main drive shaft bearings (two drops of machine oil), main drive chain, main drive motor, circulation pumps, and replenishment pumps as needed or specified by the manufacturer.

In low-volume[8] installations, the developer and filter should be discarded, the tank cleaned and filled with clean water, and the rack replaced. The next time the unit is required (after a weekend for example), the rack should be removed, the tanks drained, and fresh[9] developer installed. Perform monthly maintenance at this time. Record.

Inspect and clean mixing valve restrainers. Record.

Inspect and clean replenishment line filters. Make sure air blocks are not formed. Record.

Inspect operation and setting of the replenishment detection switches; clean if needed or readjust. Record.

Inspect and service (or forward memo) the silver reclamation device.

Review the quality control test film and processor records for the week.

Monthly

Observe safety practices.

As a continuation of the daily shutdown, drain all tanks.[10,11] Remove the developer filter, wash the tanks, rinse them, fill them, and circulate with warm water several minutes.[12] Then drain them and repeat three times.

Clean and inspect all racks and rack components, including entrance and exit crossovers and dryer rollers. Record.

Clean and inspect the main drive components.

Remove, clean, and inspect all dryer air tubes. Wipe down the dryer compartment.

Wash/clean all interior surfaces of the unit, the exterior of the tanks[13], the tubes, the motor housing or splash shields, the wires, etc.

Install a clean or new developer filter[14] (approximately 75 μm). Make sure the filter cap is tight[15] before turning on the circulation pump.

Install fresh chemicals.[16] Chemicals should be changed for convenience and not because of a deteriorated condition.

Install racks carefully.

Install water filters as needed (approximately 5 to 10 μm).

Start up according to daily start-up procedures above.

Compare before and after chemical change quality control test films and against the master when operating status is reached. Make necessary corrections.

Record all service performed, observations, and recommendations. Identify problem areas and trends. Record and review quality control test data for the month.

Flush the floor drain with drain cleaner.

Inspect the drive chain and belts while they are running. Adjust alignment (when shut down) but do not overtighten.

Perform a safelight test.

Clean the exterior surface of unit.

Quarterly

Use safety practices.

At monthly cleaning, discard the remaining chemicals in the replenishment tanks and fill with warm water. Scrub, drain, and refill with a calibrated vessel. Calibrate tanks from empty to full. Pump water through the tubing and filter, into the clean processor. Drain and refill with fresh chemicals. Check lines for air blocks.

Check the level of the feed tray, processor frame, racks, and rack support blocks. Check in all directions. Correct as needed.

Clean the dryer drive rollers, gears, and mounts. Clean the air tube springs.

Inspect the entire electrical harness, including connections, for deterioration, corrosion, looseness, etc. Correct and record.

Check the poppet valves.

Clean and/or lubricate all electrical relays and switches where possible.

Inspect and observe operation with and without the electrical signal.

Yearly

Use safety practices.

Work may be done throughout the year as an extension of monthly or quarterly duties.

Disassemble totally, inspect, renew, and rebuild each rack[17] including crossovers. Start with the developer rack. Inspect all bearings and shafts.[18]

Disassemble all motors, gearboxes, and pump heads. Clean, inspect, lubricate, or service them as needed.

Retube the unit.[19,20] This can be done piecemeal and should be done every time a pump or fitting is changed or worked on. Replace all T's, fittings, and spring clamps.

Check electrical load limits and for safety ground.

Inspect the water vacuum breaker for function.

Rebuild the mixing valve.

Rebuild the thermostats when possible.

Replace the trim gasket.

Disconnect, inspect, and clean the dryer exhaust duct.

Clean the floor drain mechanically.

Clean out header-type drain boxes.

Check the archival quality twice yearly or quarterly, especially if a cold-water processor is in use. Check at least once in the summer, once in winter.

Monitor and record ambient conditions of the film storage area for fresh film and patient films.

Clean out the dryer blower. Do not disturb weights. Check bearings.

Touch up appearance details by patching, painting, or covering with contact paper or wallpaper. Repaint where possible. Wash exterior areas.

Review processor performance: films processed (volume) versus downtime, failures, repair time, repair costs, parts volume and costs, and repeat films. Develop a plan for improvement.

Review the processor's processing consistency of quality of the product produced. Develop a plan for improvement.

Notes

1. Begin cleaning at the developer tank/rack and work toward dryer to avoid contamination in cleaning pad. Rinse the pad or sponge frequently. Plastic pads come in a variety of degrees of coarseness; many will remove rust and cut stainless steel; therefore, they are used to loosen dirt, not to remove dirt. Light, fast pressure is important. Let the warm water do most of the work.

2. A sensitometrically exposed film is a film from a special box of film that has been exposed under a controlled set of exposure (sensitization) conditions. This might be x-rays with an aluminum step wedge and a certain cassette and screen. It might be a sensitometer, which uses light and is more consistent than x-ray generators. It is simply called a quality control test film. The exposed strip must always be fed into the processor in the same direction, and this is best done by feeding the exposed area parallel to the rollers. Make the exposure at the time of processing and not in advance. The box of test film that is set aside must be protected and only used for quality control work. When the film is used up, obtain a second box and see how it compares with the first box. Record the change in emulsion number or characteristics.

3. A cleanup film must be a green unprocessed film. It could be exposed or unexposed film of any size, but scrap 14 × 17-inch film works best. Preprocessed film should not be used.

4. Wash water tanks should be self-draining so that when the water flow is restricted, the tank drains dry. This is the best method for controlling

algae growth and debris accumulation. On some units, the drain is left slightly open (flow of $\frac{1}{4}$ gallon/minute). On other units, a hole $\frac{1}{16}$ to $\frac{1}{8}$ inch in diameter is drilled in the standpipe base or the gasket is cut.

5. Pinhole leaks before a pump will cause air to be drawn into the line. Rapid oxidation follows, as well as a stiff foam that can cause further problems. Leaks after the pump cause chemicals to be blown into the hot processor cabinet, where they dry into crystals and are further distributed by the dryer. These crystals, mostly aluminum from the fixer, can do damage to films and electrical motors.

6. Glass thermometers may be filled with mercury, iodine, or alcohol. Glass breaks and cannot be calibrated easily. Mercury and iodine thermometers must never be used. Bimetallic (stem or dial) thermometers are better, usually cheaper, and may be calibrated. Electronic thermometers costing less than $70 are now available, but be sure to use stainless steel probes.

7. Eastman Kodak X-OMAT models M6-AN and M6-AW use float indicators that must be calibrated by adding a T or Y or quick-disconnect fittings at the outlet side of the flow meter (actually the flow indicator on the front of the unit). The M6-AN can also be measured by attaching a tube to the quick disconnect at the pump. Hold the tube to the same height as the flow indicator. All tests should involve priming the system plus three tests.

8. Maintenance schedules, replenishment rates, and other factors depend on the amount of use (in film volume) a processor gets. Generally, fewer problems are encountered in higher-volume units when compared with the numbers of films processed.

Processor capacity/ hour	Volume/ day	Replenish rate	Maintenance	Class
100–300	50–150	High (90–100)	Frequent (weekly)	Low
100–300	250–400	Medium (60)	Normal	Medium
100–300	500–1000	Low (50)	Frequent (weekly)	High

9. Fresh chemistry means "just made." Diluted chemistry will last about 2 weeks and should then be discarded or have substantial fresh added to it. Fresh developer added to the processor usually requires the addition of starter solution. Consult the instructions given by the chemical manufacturer. Concentrated (undiluted) chemical will last about 1 year (just like film) when stored under the same conditions of 70°F and away from direct sunlight. Avoid excessive agitation in mixing and in storage.

10. The function of the fixer is to remove all undeveloped silver halide crystals from the film. This results in dissolved silver in the fixer, termed silver-laden fixer. The silver is toxic in this form and thus must be removed prior to putting the used fixer down the drain. Thus, we have silver recovery for ecological reasons as well as for the more obvious economic reasons. The fixer in the processor at cleaning time also is rich in silver (normally 0.6 troy ounces/gallon) and must be considered. If the fixer tank is drained in some units, the silver-laden fixer will miss the recovery device. In other units, when the fixer is drained it passes through the recovery device but the flow is so great that no recovery takes place and silver is lost. In both cases, the silver-laden fixer should be collected and processed separately.

11. When racks are removed from solution, immediately flush with running water for several minutes to remove hazardous chemicals and to prevent chemicals from drying out and producing gum and crystals. This is also true of pumps and the circulation system: Flush it as soon as it is drained.

12. On some processors, when the tank is drained, the pump head and some of the tubing are still filled with chemicals. This chemical trap must be blown out, flushed out, or hosed out. Those units that have complete draining through the pump head also usually have contained heat exchangers that benefit from flushing.

13. Stainless steel tanks will rust if held in contact with another steel that rusts. Therefore, steel wool pads must never be used, and dropped screws etc. must be immediately retrieved. However, most stainless steel tanks rust from the outside in as a result of chemical splatters that dry out. On very dirty exteriors, carefully remove excess debris but be careful about removing all debris unless you are prepared to epoxy hundreds of pinholes.

14. Air must be removed from the filter. Soak the filter in warm water or in the developer replenishment tank prior to use.

15. The developer filter cap must be tight, and this puts a set into the gasket. Turning the gasket over each time will prolong its life. If an older gasket (which has not been turned) starts to leak, turn it over. Each time the gasket is turned, inspect it.

16. Add fixer to a clean processor first; if any splashes into the clean, dry developer tank, it will be easily seen and flushed out. Always add developer second. Starter can be poured in on top of the developer, because when the rack is replaced it will adequately mix the starter into the developer.

17. Make sure the developer rack and associated crossovers are always in perfect condition. If a damaged roller is found in the fixer rack during yearly breakdown, use a developer rack roller and put the new roller in the developer rack. Crossovers are often interchange-

able but must never be interchanged. To prevent this, label with an etching tool, tape, or paint.

18. A shaft will often be worn, grooved, galled, etc.; replacing the bearing and not the shaft is a worthless act. Where shafts are reasonably good but the bearing is worn on one side (egg shaped), the bearing can be cleaned and rotated 180° without the need for a new one. This is also true of roller studs.

19. Spring-type hose clamps are usually of the Corbin type and are designed for one-time use. When removing them, always wear safety glasses and use only hose-clamp pliers. Apply pressure and move down the tubing; release pressure as soon as possible. Do not reuse or replace these clamps. Install screw-type strap clamps. Corbin clamps can explode and should be treated with extreme caution.

20. When retubing, look for, remove, and reinstall line restrictors, which are usually 1-inch-long plastic plugs with about a ⅛-inch hole in the center. Tubing dries out with age and requires annual replacement. Usually called Tygon (brand name of Norton Plastics Company), it is flexible polyvinylchloride (PVC). Use ⅛-inch wall material of any brand, general grade. Stepping up or down or fitting tubing to a pump or tank fitting of the same diameter is best done by using a sleeve of tubing of the next ¼-inch larger size.

General

In general, in the production of the useful, visible image, all directives and controls should be coordinated by the film manufacturer and not by the chemistry or processor manufacturer. Film will work under a variety of conditions, but not with the same degree of flexibility as the chemicals or processor. In this regard, processor manufacturer recommendations can only be used as guidelines, even for the same manufacturer's film and chemistry.

Correct storage for film and chemicals (in storage, in darkroom/light room, and after processing) is 70°F, 60% relative humidity (RH), film on edge, first-in-first-out (FIFO) storage system, good lighting and ventilation (ceilings are hotter than floors), away from direct sunlight or radiators, no bumping or jostling of the chemicals, and a record system.

Record everything in a file or laboratory-type book. It will document and prove what you have done and will direct you in the future.

Systems cleaners are hazardous to people, to chemistry, and to the ecology. They should be used less frequently and only to clean out tanks and circulation systems. They should never be used on racks or have racks soaking in them. When used on racks, the rollers absorb and trap small amounts, resulting in lost film quality and increased production of dirt in the developer tank. Granular types must be fully dissolved before pumps are turned on.

Canister-type (metallic displacement) silver recovery units (also called buckets) are a primary cause of drain clogging due to an accumulation of iron oxide particles flushed from the unit. This type of unit should not be used, but where used, increase the frequency of the chemical treatment of the drain.

Processor-Processing Maintenance Schedules

Daily

- Start up.
  Check all solution levels.
  Check the replenishment tank quantity.
  Inspect transport running.
  Work the microswitches.
  Clean the feed tray.
  Check for leaks, general inspection.
  Wash the crossovers.
  Check the chemical color.
  Record observations, work, and recommendations.
- At run status (beginning of shift)
  Feed several green cleanup films.
  Run a sensitometric test film and make a visual comparison to a standard. If they do not match acceptably, check processor time and temperatures.
  Correct the conditions to produce acceptable results.
  Record observations and work conclusions, including a sensitometric plot.
- Midday (middle of shift)
  Clean the feed tray.
  Inspect general parameters (replenishment, temperature, feed time, etc.).
  Run a sensitometric control, make visual comparison; correct if needed.
  Record observations.
- After periods of 1 hour or more on standby
  Clean the feed tray.
  Run several green cleanup films and/or clean crossovers.
  Run a sensitometric strip.
  Record.
- Running serial film or cine film
  Run a sensitometric strip first. If it is okay, process work film.

Run a sensitometric film afterward to verify consistent processing or to indicate a need for change prior to next run.
Record.

- Shutdown (end of shift)

Run a sensitometric strip. Compare with the standard. Record.
Remove and wash the crossovers.
Wipe out inside processor all splatter, spills, etc.
Inspect generally.
Leave fume controls, splash guards, and crossovers on top of processor. Cover with a towel.
Crack open 1 to 2 inches at the top cover of the processor.
Record.

- Other—general

Train operators to be aware of and responsive to sounds, smell, vibrations of processor, the way film feeds, and any unusual occurrences throughout the day. Establish direct and easy communication and record these observations.
Restrict processor monitoring, sensitometric evaluation, jam clearing, etc. to one person per area or processor.
Sensitometric tests are designed to show if a unit is performing correctly within predetermined limits. If the processing is out of limits or trending toward out of limits, corrective action must be taken or unacceptable radiographs will result.
Sensitometric data plots can be posted near the processor. Wear safety goggles and other protective equipment at all times. Always use safe working procedures, such as posting signs and restricting nonworkers from the area during work.
Never soak rollers or racks in systems cleaners.

Weekly

Remove the developer rack and hose it down with hot water; inspect and replace it.

Check the replenishment rate for accuracy (the volume with tank full, half full, empty) and reproducibility (same volume with same volume of replenisher tank at the same pump setting).

Check to see if the replenishment pump, thermostat, and mixing valve settings have been altered.

Verify or recalibrate all thermometers, including the one on mixing valve using an external calibrated bimetallic stem thermometer.

Check the temperatures of all solutions with calibrated thermometers.

Check the developer immersion time and feed rate (this allows calculation of transport rate).

Lubricate the main drive shaft bearings, dryer drive mechanism, and motors with fittings for light oil.

Clean and grease the worm gears on the main drive shaft.

Clean and relubricate the main drive chain.

Check the alignment and tension of the main drive chain and dryer drive belt.

Review weekly sensitometry trends.

Quarterly

Drain all chemicals from the processor and replenishment tank, scrub out, rinse, fill with warm water, and pump.

Calibrate (or verify) the markings on the replenishment tanks from empty to completely filled.

Check that the processor, support bars, racks, and feed tray are level.

Record.

Biannually

Use a system cleaner to clean the heat exchanger in the developer section only if a problem is anticipated. Fill the tank, add cleaner, circulate for 5 minutes, drain, and flush three times.

Annually (spread work throughout the year)

Disassemble each rack and crossover completely; inspect and replace parts. Especially inspect stud holes, studs bearings, and shafts and for signs of wear.

Disassemble the main drive shaft and components; clean and inspect bearings.

Replace all tubing.

Record.

Review all records; develop program for following year.

If a densitometer is available, read, plot, calculate, and record sensitometric values: D_{max}, contrast, speed, and base plus fog (B + F).

Record all observations and work performed.

Monthly

- Twice monthly
  Remove deep racks and scrub them with hot water and a plastic cleaning pad such as Pako Pad, Dobie, or Scotch Brite. Inspect and replace them. Clean the master roller in the turnaround assembly.

Clean up all spills and splatters under tanks.

Record observations and work.

- Once monthly

Clean dryer air tubes, rollers, and compartment.

Change out all chemicals.

Change the developer and water filter; clean replenishment and mixing valve strainers.

Scrub tanks, rinse, fill them with warm water, and circulate for 5 minutes. Drain and rinse. Make sure all fluid is out of the pumps.

Make any necessary repairs.

Refill with fresh chemicals.

Record observations and work.

Review records for the month with the staff. Training could also be included.

Records

Records provide information to help make decisions, just as a patient's medical history often is necessary to help the physician understand a medical problem. The more records the better, but they must be meaningful and easy to use. One worker might prefer to maintain a series of charts; another would choose to keep a file of notes, cleaning schedules, etc.; and a third might find a diary more beneficial. There is no single correct method, but the wrong method is not to keep records. In science, record books are kept like a diary. The researcher dates an entry, titles the project, and records every detail. At the end of the project, the entry is initialled or signed by the worker. Of course the best records are of no value unless they are reviewed and/or summarized periodically. Consider the problems someone might encounter if they were to consult another worker's records in their absence. Would they be able to find complete information? A separate diary or file should be kept on each processor. Include the amount of time spent on each job. Make notes to yourself or to other workers to check certain problem areas and institute a policy to encourage all workers to look for these notes. Make the records available to service personnel and sales personnel who are troubleshooting, servicing, or consulting. Simply put, do the records tell you the condition of the processor at any given moment? They should.

Economics

As film prices change, as silver prices change, and as the general economy changes, the elements of the following discussion will probably change but the concept will not. Historically, for a dollar's worth of unexposed green film, about $5 in radiation, personnel (technologist, aids, secretaries, porters), and overhead must be expended to form the latent image. The function of processing is to form the useful, visible image, and this costs about $.30. This breaks down to about $.05 for developer, $.05 for fixer, and $.20 for equipment amortization, repairs, parts, utilities, and service or maintenance contract. Clearly, chemicals are the least expensive component, and a good quality should be purchased from a reliable source. The single largest expense is personnel, which often consumes 75% of the budget. When the production of a department is flowing smoothly, there is a return on investment of about $10 gross. However, should a technologist have to repeat a film, the return on investment is cut in half and the result is a loss of about $10 on one exam. Repeats are expensive but normally account for only 3 to 7% of all films. A repeat analysis should be initiated. Contact the film companies about this program and also about cost analysis programs. It is important to understand that medicine is business. Sound business principles to guide the operation of the department are a partner to technical principles.

Parts Lists

Each institution should have an allocation of 10% of a processor's purchase price devoted to spare parts, which are kept replenished as they are used. This parts supply will cost from $500 to $1600 for most processors. Pako and Du Pont offer parts cabinets for common failure parts that are well worth the investment. Spare parts should be kept and inventoried at the institution even if a service person does the installation. Most parts are the small components such as fuses, gears, pins, springs, switches, etc. Larger items such as pumps are very expensive, but to buy an extra pump head is inexpensive, and this part usually breaks down before the motor does. If an institution has more than two processors, then a spare main drive motor, replenishment pump, and circulation pump should be purchased. An annual allocation (amortization-replacement fund) should be provided to rebuild the developer rack and to eventually purchase a complete extra rack by the third year. Any replacement rollers should be placed in the developer rack and the older rollers used to replace damaged rollers in the fixer and wash.

Chapter 8

Troubleshooting Guides

The more one has to troubleshoot, the less effective is the preventive maintenance schedule or program. But once the trouble exists, how does one start to unravel the problem? Start at the problem and look for clues. For instance, a jammed film may be due to a transport problem but is usually the result of a failure of the developer hardener. Keep records so that future problems can be cross-checked with past problems. It serves no purpose to keep fixing the same problem. The objective is consistent quality (quality control). Most guides are designed to provide help in finding answers but also are an educational tool to help educate the users. Guides are often used several times, and the worker then files the guide away and proceeds on basic knowledge learned.

Processor Problem-Solving Guide

Transport Problems

Sheet Film Jams

1. Turn off the drive motor or the power. Look inside and try to save as many films as possible.
2. Remove the crossover rack ahead of the pileup.

3. Remove the films at this point. Put them in a tray of water to keep them from sticking together.
4. Clear the film. If a rack is wet from solution, turn off the circulation pump for that solution.
   CAUTION: If the fixer rack must be removed, be careful not to drop fixer into the developer.
   Remove the rack where the jam occurred and examine it for the cause of the problem.
5. Feed the removed film into the rack nearest the point of jamming, to complete the processing cycle.

Film Twisting or Turning in Processing Section

1. Be sure the crossovers are seated properly.
2. Be sure the crossovers and solution racks are square.
3. Check for burrs on the guide plates in the racks.
4. Check for stretched springs on the racks, which would lead to uneven roller pressure.

Film Jams in the Processing Section

1. See causes under "Film Twisting or Turning," above.
2. Be sure two films were not fed one on top of the other.
3. Films shorter than 10.2 cm (4 inches) cannot be reliably fed without a leader tab.
4. Check for badly stretched roller springs on the racks.
5. Check for broken or bound end bearings on the rack rollers.
6. Check for broken teeth on the rack gears.
7. Be sure all gears are meshed and not just riding on top of the teeth.
8. Check for worn gears or worms.
9. Check for chemical deposits on the racks.
10. Check for warped rollers.
11. Check for a temperature or chemical problem that is causing film to be tacky.
12. Check for a loose guide plate.

Film Jams in the Dryer

1. Be sure the exit crossover is seated properly.
2. Be sure the dryer rollers are seated properly.
3. If the dryer drive has stopped, check the connecting gears.
4. Check for any conditions causing the film to dry improperly: dryer temperature too low, exhaust inefficiency, low replenishment, temperatures too high, high ambient humidity, etc.
5. Make sure air tubes face the correct direction.

Lengthwise Scratches on the Film

1. Check for encrusted chemical deposits on the racks, particularly at or above the solution level and feed tray.
2. Check for burns on the guide plates in the racks.
3. Check to see if a roller is not turning because of broken gear teeth, etc.
4. Check for reversed or out-of-position guide shoes.

Pressure Marks on Films

1. Check for foreign material or rough spots on the roller.
2. Check for a roller that is warped or too tight.
3. Consider developer hardener failure; replace the developer.

Excessive Gear Damage

The sun gear on the drive end of the racks may have gotten chewed up.

1. The rack may have been dropped into the tank too hard, bending the indexing pins. With a hammer, carefully drive down the pins until they are parallel with the rest of the rack.
2. If the plastic and steel gears do not mesh, bend the rail slightly. There should be very little play in the gears.
3. Be sure that the gears are kept clean.

Electrical Problems

Motor Starting Relays

The circulation pump motors are started by current-type motor starting relays. When voltage is applied to the motor (by closing the heat or cool switch), the first rush of current through the motor main winding and starting relay coil closes the normally open (NO) relay contacts. This allows current to flow in the motor starter winding and starts the motor. As the motor speed increases, the current drops in the main winding and relay coil, opening the relay contacts to disconnect the starter winding. The motor is then in its normal condition.

If defective, the relay should be replaced as a unit. When installing the new relay, check the wiring diagrams for color coding of the wires and position.

Developer Switch Motor does not Operate with Heat or Cool Switch Depressed

1. If one switch activates the pump motor but the other does not, either the later switch is defective or there is an error in the wiring to it.
2. If neither switch activates the motor, turn the developer thermostat all

the way down to energize the cool solenoid valve. If the solenoid is not energized, trace the power supply to the machine and up to the heat and cool switches.

3. If, however, the solenoid is energized in step 2, trace the wiring to the motor and motor starter.
4. If the wiring appears correct, replace the motor starter. If this still does not solve the problem, replace the motor.

Fixer Pump Motor Does Not Operate
With Circulation-Replenishment Switch Depressed

1. Feed a sheet of film into the machine. If the replenisher pump motors are activated, the power supply is correct through the circulation-re-plenishment switch. Check the wiring to the fixer circulation pump motor and motor starter. If the wiring seems correct, replace the motor starter. If this still does not solve the problem, replace the motor.

Replenisher Pump Does Not Run

If a replenisher pump does not run when the circulation-replenishment switch is on and a replenisher microswitch is depressed and

1. If only one pump motor does not run, trace the wiring to that motor. If the wiring seems correct, replace the motor.
2. If neither motor runs, trace the wiring to the coil of relay K4 (if included) and to its NO contacts. If the wiring seems correct, be sure the replenisher microswitch is being fully depressed. If it is not, readjust it.
3. If the microswitch is being activated, jump across its terminals. If this energizes relay K4, replace the switch; if not, replace the relay.

Drive Motor Does Not Run with Drive Switch Depressed

1. If there is power to the rest of the machine, check the wiring to the switch and drive motor to see if it is correct. If it seems correct, check the switch and drive motor.

Tempering Problems

Developer Temperature Fluctuates

1. Check the switch and fuses for the immersion heaters.
2. See "Circulation/Filtration Problems" for a possible cause of impaired circulation.
3. Be sure that the incoming cold water to the heat exchanger is adequate and at least 5° colder than the desired tempered water temperature.
4. Check the developer thermometer for function and accuracy.

5. Replace the developer thermostat.
6. Replace the thermocouple sensing element.
7. Replace the immersion heater(s).
8. Check the solenoid valve when used.

Solenoid Valve Leaks

1. Disassemble the valve as outlined above and clean the valve seat and ball. Use crocus cloth, emery cloth, etc. to remove any scale or rust deposits on the seating surface.
2. If the seating surface is damaged or the plunger or spring is worn, replace the valve.

Solenoid Valve Does Not Open or Close Properly

1. Disassemble the valve and check for foreign matter.
2. Be sure the plunger is not binding the tube.
3. Check the action of the spring.

Other

Film and Chemistry Problems

Problems with film and chemistry and the solutions to these problems will vary with the material being used. For most of the following problems, therefore, also consult with the film and chemical technical sales representatives.

Incorrect Film Density

1. Check the mixing procedure for the developer and replenisher to be sure that they conform to the procedure supplied with the particular batch of chemicals you are using. Mixing instructions can change from batch to batch, and the only instructions that should be used are those enclosed with the chemicals.
2. Check the replenishment rate. If the change in density has been gradual, the problem may be over- or underreplenishing.
3. Check the causes of over- or underreplenishment listed under "Replenishment System Problems."
4. Do not use the developer beyond the time recommended by the manufacturer.
5. Be sure the developer has not been contaminated with fixer or foreign chemicals.
6. Be sure the developer temperature is as recommended by the film manufacturer.
7. Make sure the processing tank is at the correct level.
8. Make sure there is adequate agitation.

Mottling

Mottling of the film is most often caused by too high a developer concentration. Check with the developer supplier and/or perform a specific gravity test using a hydrometer.

Streaking

Streaks on the film are most often caused by weak developer and/or weak fixer. Check the replenishment rate: Change the solutions if necessary. See also the information on drying streaks under "Air/Dryer Problems."

Yellow Smudges

Yellow smudges are often caused by exhausted fixer.

Film Does Not Clear

If the film does not clear, the fixer concentration is probably too low, is contaminated, or is old or appears so because of a failure of the developer hardener to control swelling.

Pi Lines

Pi lines on the film are normal with fresh chemicals and should disappear after a short run. Run green film to clean rollers.

Dirt on the Film

Dirt on the film usually comes from the water supply. If there is a filter in the water supply line, change the cartridge; if the water is not filtered, it would be wise to install one. Too little agitation or flow of any solution will contribute to dirt accumulation. Check for algae in the wash tank. Check for dust in the dryer.

Drying

If films stick to the rollers in the dryer, they have not been properly hardened. There are several possible causes.
1. Be sure you are using chemicals that are designed for roller processing and that are compatible with the brand of film being used.
2. The fixer may be exhausted or underreplenished.
3. The developer may be diluted, underreplenished, or old.
4. The solution temperatures may be too high for the film.
5. The solutions may be contaminated or may have been improperly mixed.
6. Check the causes of inadequate solution circulation listed under "Circulation/Filtration System Problems."

7. The wash may be inadequate. Check the causes of inadequate wash water flow in the mixing-valve instruction manual.
8. There may be a dryer malfunction.

Processor Troubleshooting Checklist

Transport System

Roller subsystem components (film-handling problems)
- Rollers: size, hardness, driven, nondriven, squeegee
- Roller pins, studs, shafts, bearings
- Guide shoes: adjustable, nonadjustable
- Deflector plates, wires, bars
- Face plates
- Tie bars, support bars
- Feed tray

Motor subsystem components (speed, drive problems)
- Electrical power supply
- Switch, fuses, relays
- Motor: brushes, controllers, gears
- Gears, sprockets, pulleys
- Chains, belts
- Bearings
- Shafts

Transport Problems are Caused by

1. Misaligned gears, sprockets
2. Misaligned chains, belts
3. Misaligned turnarounds, crossovers
4. Misaligned racks
5. Misaligned guide shoes, deflector plates
6. Misaligned drive shafts
7. Misaligned support bars
8. Misaligned feed tray
9. Worn, broken gears or sprockets
10. Worn, broken chains or belts
11. Worn, broken bearings or shafts
12. Tension springs too tight or too loose
13. Roller gear ends loose
14. Dryer drive misalignment
15. Roller studs binding
16. Time-delay-on-feed too short
17. Dirty rollers
18. Fuses, breakers, or protectors
19. Slipping gears or sprockets
20. Slipping chains or belts

21. Broken electrical conductor, terminal, or connector
22. Damaged switch
23. Electrical power source
24. Drive motor gears damaged
25. Drive motor starter circuit damaged
26. Drive motor run circuit damaged
27. Damaged rollers
28. Damaged drive shafts
29. Chemical failure: developer, fixer, or hardeners
30. Film characteristics: size, type, sides
31. Lubrication
33. Cleanliness
34. Film-feeding procedure

Transport problems	Common cause	Or check these causes
Film jams	1–8	1–17, 19, 20, 24, 27–34
Abrasions	1–4	3–5, 7–15, 17, 19, 20, 27–33
Overlapped films	16, 34	3–5, 7–16, 19, 20, 27, 28, 30, 32, 34
Cocked films	8, 34	3–5, 8, 11–15, 17, 27–28, 31–34
Detector switch activation	8, 22	1, 2, 5–13, 15, 17, 19, 20, 22, 27–28
Unusual noise	1, 2	1, 2, 4, 6, 7, 9–15, 19–20, 24, 27, 28, 31–34
Film dropping in dryer	14, 32	1, 2, 4, 6, 9–15, 19–20, 27, 28, 30, 32
Film retained in dryer	29	1, 2, 4, 7, 9–12, 14–17, 19, 20, 27, 28, 29–33
Increased density	27, 31	1, 3–5, 9–15, 19, 20, 27–29, 31, 33
Decreased density		4, 14, 23, 29–32
Rapid gear, sprocket wear	31, 33	1–7, 14, 15, 17, 19, 20, 27, 28, 29, 31–33
Component not turning	1, 9	1–7, 9–15, 18–28, 31–33
Scratches	5, 29	1–15, 19, 20, 27–34
Gelatin pick-off deposit	17, 19	3–7, 9–15, 17, 19, 20, 27–30, 32, 33
Pressure marks	4	3–7, 9–13, 15, 17, 19, 20, 27, 29, 33, 34

Replenishment System

Components

- Detector switch (microswitch)
- Detector assembly: airflow, rollers
- Main switch, fuses, relays
- Pump: head, motor, gearbox
- Lines: tubing, fittings
- Gauges: flow indicators, meters
- Tanks: outside processor
- Check valves
- Needle valves
- Filters

Replenishment Problems are Caused by

1. Detector switch malfunction
2. Detector switch adjustment
3. Detector assembly malfunction
4. Cleanliness of detector assembly, switch
5. Electrical supply
6. Pump setting
7. Pump accuracy
8. Pump reproducibility
9. Pump leak
10. Pump malfunction
11. Lines kinked, blocked
12. Lines: air leak, air block
13. Lines: solution leak
14. Lines: fittings damaged
15. Gauges not calibrated
16. Filters or strainers clogged
17. Tanks not calibrated
18. Check valves stuck
19. Check valves deteriorated
20. Check valves installed incorrectly
21. Adjustment valve failure
22. Replenishment tanks empty
23. Frequency of mix
24. Absence of floating lids
25. Water supply problems

Replenishment problems	*Common cause*	*Or check these causes*
Chemistry volume low	6–8	1–24
Chemistry volume high	6–8, 18	1, 2, 4, 6–8, 15, 17–20, 23
Chemistry activity low	6–8, 18	1–24
Chemistry activity high	6–8, 18	1, 2, 6–8, 15, 17–20, 23
Increased density	6–8	1–4, 6–8, 15, 17–21, 23
Unclear film	6–8	1–24
Unwashed film (mixing valve)	6–8	1–24
Film not dry	25	1–24
Scratches, abrasions	6–8	1–24
Film jams	6–8	1–24
Decreased density	6–8	1–24
Chemical breakdown	6–8	1–24
High consumption	6, 24	1–24
Leaks	13, 14	9, 11–14, 16, 12–21
Variable sensitometry	7, 8	1, 4, 7, 8, 17

Electrical System

Components

- Power supply
- Lock-out box, fuses, terminals
- Processor switches
- Processor relays
- Processor terminals
- Processor fuses, circuit breakers
- Motor protectors
- Motors: pump, drive
- Heaters: developer, dryer
- Indicator lights
- Thermostats: developer, dryer
- Conductors

Electrical Problems are Caused by

1. No supply at source
2. Half normal supply (1 line)
3. Wrong phase

 4. Variable supply
 5. Line voltage fluctuation
 6. Loaded line (elevator etc. on same line)
 7. Fuses burned
 8. Fuses corroded
 9. Fuses broken
10. Wrong size fuse
11. Circuit breaker blown (open)
12. Circuit breaker broken
13. Relay stuck closed
14. Relay stuck open
15. Burned contacts
16. Welded contacts
17. Bent contacts, rocker plates
18. Broken switch open
19. Broken switch closed
20. Jammed switch open
21. Jammed switch closed
22. Motor starter switch defective
23. Motor starter windings burned or shorted
24. Motor running windings burned or shorted
25. Heater element burned or shorted
26. Thermostat switch malfunction
27. Indicator light burned out
28. Loose connections
29. Short circuit in conductors
30. Corroded connectors
31. Heat
32. Lack of lubrication

Electrical problems	Common cause	Or check these causes
Nothing runs	1–3	1–3, 6, 11, 12, 14, 15, 17, 18, 20, 29, 30
Drive motor won't start	22, 23	1–9, 11, 12, 14, 15, 17, 18, 20, 22, 23, 28–32
Drive motor starts, won't run	24	24
Drive motor manual start, will run	22, 23	1–9, 11, 12, 15, 17, 18, 20, 22, 23, 28, 30, 32
Pump motor won't start	22, 23	1–9, 11, 12, 14, 17, 20, 22, 23, 28, 29, 30, 31, 33

Electrical problems	Common cause	Or check these causes
Pump motor won't run	24	24
Motor speed changes	4, 32	3–6, 24, 28, 32
Motors fail annually	4, 32	2–6, 10, 30, 31, 32
No circulation	22, 26, 32	1–9, 11, 12, 14, 15, 17, 18, 20, 22–24, 26, 28–32
No heat	7, 25, 26	1–9, 11–12, 14, 15, 17, 18, 20, 25–30
Too much heat	10, 13, 26	3–5, 10, 13, 16, 17, 19, 21, 26, 27
Too little heat	26	2–9, 11, 12, 14, 26–31
Insufficient replenishment	14	2–9, 14, 17, 24, 28–32
Heater won't turn off	13	10–13, 16, 17, 19, 21, 26, 29
Motor won't turn off	13, 16, 21	13, 16, 17, 19, 21, 29
Insulation burned	6, 13	3–6, 10, 29–31
Insulation crumbling	6, 13	3–6, 10, 29–31

Circulation/Filtration System

Circulation Components
- Electrical power supply
- Switch, fuses, relays
- Pump motor starter
- Pump motor
- Heat exchanger
- Tubing, fittings

Filtration Components
- Filter type
- Filter size

Circulation/Filtration Problems are Caused by

1. Line voltage fluctuations
2. Pumps not lubricated
3. Failure of pump motor thermostat
4. Burned motor starter
5. Burned motor starter windings
6. Dirty magnets, shafts
7. Worn bearings
8. Loose pump/motor linkage
9. Warped pump head

10. Leaking pump head
11. Leaking tubing
12. Leaking fittings
13. Air blockage of pumps
14. Air blockage of filters
15. Block tubing
16. Improper flow, i.e., backward
17. Filter clogged
18. Filter caked
19. Filter channels
20. Filter size too small
21. Filter size too large
22. Filter missing
23. Heat exchanger leaking
24. Heat exchanger clogged
25. Dirty pump
26. Defective switch

Circulation/filtration problems	Common cause	Or check these causes
No circulation	4, 17	2–18, 20, 25, 26, 27
Reduced flow	26	1–18, 29, 24–27
Variable flow	1–3	1–3, 6–9, 26
Pump not running	2, 3	1–5, 7, 9, 13–18, 20, 25, 26, 27
Pump okay, no flow	13, 14	10–18, 20, 25
Pump motor won't start	3, 4	1–5, 27
Pump runs after manual start	4, 5	4, 5
Very loud, noisy pump	6, 26	6–9, 13, 26
Leaks at pump	9	9–12, 16
General leaks	10	10–18, 20
Foam	13, 14	9–14, 19, 21, 23
Increased temperature of chemistry	25, 17	9–18, 20, 25
Frequent filter changes, i.e., weekly	20	18, 18, 20, 24–27

Circulation/filtration problems	Common cause	Or check these causes
Lower density	2, 3	1–18, 20, 24–27
Uncleared films	2, 3	1–18, 20, 24–27
Reduced or no replenishment	17	11, 12, 14, 17, 18
Dirt on films	21	17, 19, 21, 26

Temperature Control System

Components

- Thermostat
- Thermometers
- Switch, fuses, relays
- Water supply
- Electrical power supply

- Heaters
- Indicator lights
- Circulation pump
- Mixing valve (if used)
- Heat exchanger

Temperature problems are caused by

1. Electrical power fluctuations
2. Water supply fluctuations
3. Loss of cold water
4. Loss of hot water
5. Loss of volume
6. Loss of pressure
7. Mixing-valve malfunction
8. Clogged filters, strainers
9. Clogged heat exchanger
10. Clogged tubing
11. Thermostat stuck open
12. Thermostat stuck closed
13. Thermostat uncalibrated
14. Thermometer uncalibrated
15. Thermometer broken
16. Heater broken
17. Heater relay stuck open
18. Heater relay stuck closed
19. Indicator light burned out
20. No circulation
21. Switch or fuse failure

Temperature problems	Cause	Or check these causes
Decreased temperature/ decreased density	11	1, 2, 4–7, 11, 13–17, 19–21
Increased temperature/ increased density	3, 18	1–3, 5–10, 12–15, 18–21
Unclear films	3, 4	3–7
Unwashed films	3, 4	1–15
Undried films	17	11, 13–17, 19–21
Streaks on films	20	8–10, 20
Unequal development	8, 9, 20	1–10, 20
Unequal clearing	10, 20	1–10, 20
Unequal washing	7, 9, 20	1–10, 20
Unequal drying	16, 20	1–10, 16, 20
Temperature fluctuations	1, 2	1, 2, 7–10, 13, 14, 20
Developer gets hotter, heater off	2	2, 3, 5–7, 19
Developer does not heat	2, 21	1, 2, 4–11, 13–17, 19–21
Indicator light cycles on/off slowly	20	8–10, 13, 20
Hot water heats developer	7	2, 3, 5–10

Dryer System

Components
- Electrical supply
- Main switch, fuses, relays
- Blower/motor
- Heater(s)
- Thermostat
- Thermometer
- Safety thermostat
- Indicator light

- Exhaust
- Sheaves (pulleys, belts)
- Receiver bin
- Air tubes

Dryer Problems are Caused by

1. Electrical supply fluctuations
2. Insufficient electricity
3. Broken (open) switch, relay, or fuse
4. Broken (closed) switch, relay, or fuse
5. Stuck switch or relay
6. Blower fins clogged with dirt
7. Blower bearings worn or broken
8. Blower drive belt misaligned
9. Blower drive belt broken
10. Motor starter windings burned
11. Motor starter relay broken
12. Motor running windings burned
13. Motor circuit breaker open
14. Heater burned out
15. One of heaters burned out
16. Thermostat stuck closed
17. Thermostat stuck open
18. Safety thermostat broken or open
19. Setting on safety thermostat too high
20. Thermostat not calibrated
21. Thermometer not functioning
22. Indicator light broken
23. Air tubes dirty
24. Air tubes installed wrong
25. Exhaust tube too small
26. Exhaust tube blocked
27. Exhaust too small
28. Exhaust too great
29. Room intake air too cool
30. Rollers dirty
31. Rollers allow film slippage
32. Squeegee roller function
33. Developer depleted
34. Fixer depleted
35. No wash water
36. Transport speed too fast
37. Ambient conditions

Drying problems	Common cause	Or check these causes
Overall wet, cool, soft films	3, 17, 19, 33, 34	1–3, 5–15, 17–21, 23–27
Above, trailing edge	15, 33, 34	1, 2, 6–8, 15, 19–21, 23–27, 29–34, 36
Film cool, barely dry	15, 19, 20, 33	1, 2, 6–8, 15, 19–21, 23–34
Film hot, damp	19, 20, 37	6–10, 15, 19–21, 23–27, 30–34, 36, 37
Overall mist, warm, hard films	27	6, 25, 28, 37
Above, trailing edge	27	6, 25–28, 37
6th to 10th film becomes damp	27, 33	19–22, 25–30, 33, 34, 37
14 × 17 dry; 8 × 10 damp	31	31
8 × 10 dry; 14 × 17 damp	3, 17, 18, 33, 34	1–3, 5–15, 17–21, 23–27
Serial films become damper	27, 33	19–22, 25–30, 33, 34, 37
Marginal drying, high heat	19, 20, 25, 28	15, 18–28, 30–37
Water spots	32, 33	6, 10, 14, 15, 17–21, 30–34
Crosshatch pattern	6, 30, 33	6, 10, 15, 16, 19–27
Waveform pattern	19, 20	4–6, 10, 15, 16, 19–27
Baked, glossy surface	19, 20	6, 16, 19, 20–22
Light area surface	23, 24	23, 24
Jams	31, 33	3, 6–14, 17–37
Film cocking	31, 33	31, 33
Dirt on films	30	23, 24, 30, 33, 34
No heat	3, 14	1–3, 5, 9–12, 17–22, 28, 29, 37
No air	9, 10, 11	1–3, 5–13, 23, 24

Sensitometeric Problem-Solving Flow Chart

The flow chart on the following pages presents a logical sequence to try to locate the specific cause of a sensitometric problem. This chart deals with the problem of increased density and is only one example. These are four adverse sensitometric conditions possible:

- Increased density
- Decreased density
- Increased contrast
- Decreased contrast

Each chart works the same way, and in many cases they are similar, thus only this one example is provided.

At the beginning, upper left-hand part of page, a question is asked. The question asked represents the most common cause of this problem. The least common causes will be found at the extreme distance from this point in either the horizontal or vertical planes. If you find you can answer "yes" to the question, then proceed to define the cause further. If you answer "no," then follow that course until a "yes" answer fits.

The pages are individually coded, so a wall chart may be constructed if desired.

Guide to Following Chart Pages

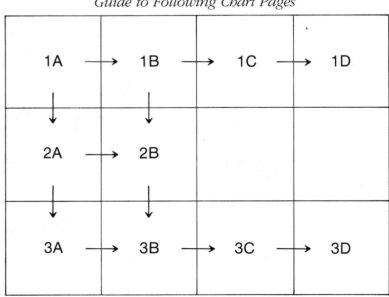

CHART 1-A

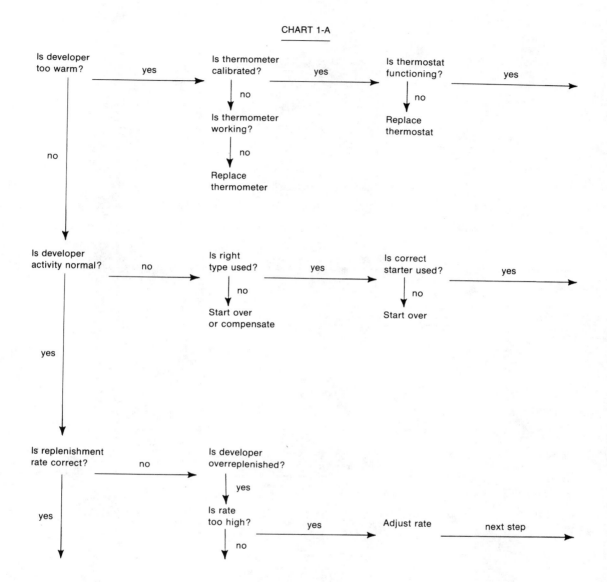

CHART 1-B

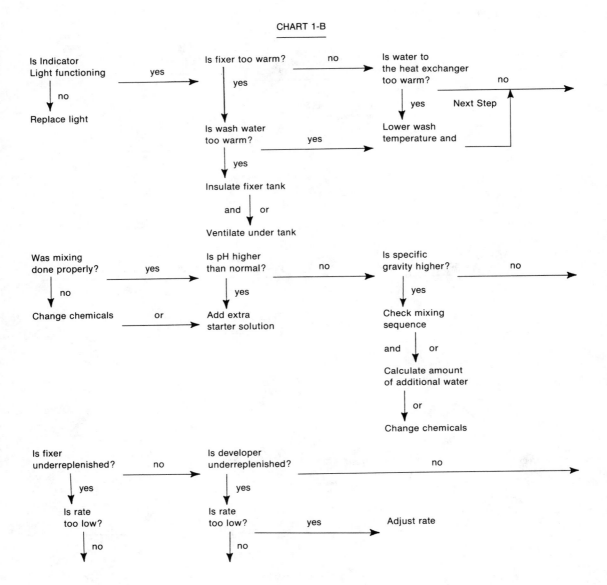

CHART 1-C

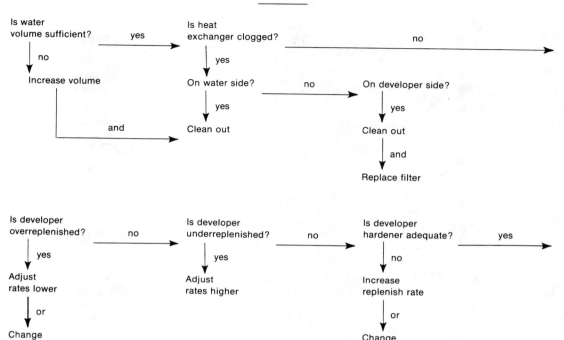

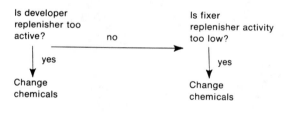

CHART 1-D

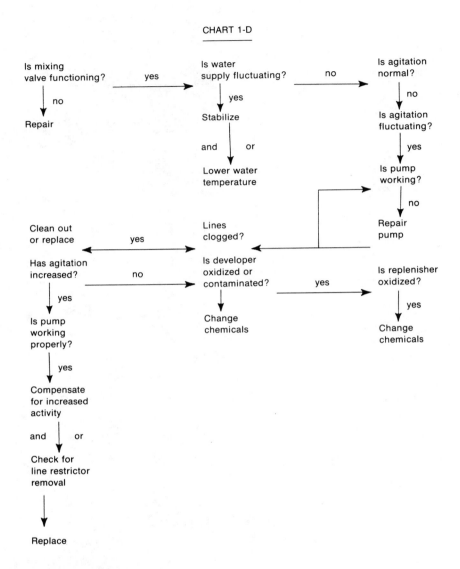

Is mixing
valve functioning?   —— yes ——>   Is water
supply fluctuating?   —— no ——>   Is agitation
normal?

| no | yes | no

Repair   Stabilize   Is agitation
fluctuating?

                                          and | or | yes

                                          Lower water
                                          temperature   Is pump
working?

                                                                                       | no

Clean out
or replace   <—— yes ——   Lines
clogged?   <——————   Repair
pump

Has agitation
increased?   —— no ——>   Is developer
oxidized or
contaminated?   —— yes ——>   Is replenisher
oxidized?

| yes | | yes

Is pump
working
properly?   Change
chemicals   Change
chemicals

| yes

Compensate
for increased
activity

and | or

Check for
line restrictor
removal

|

Replace

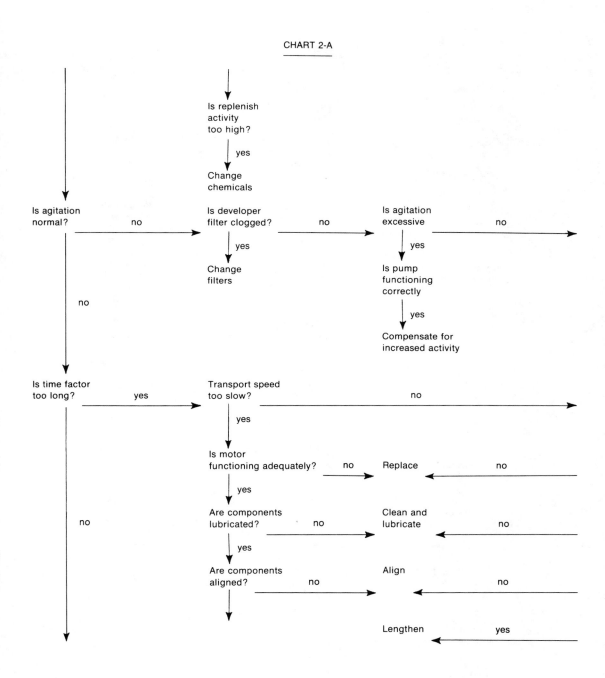

CHART 2-A

CHART 2-B

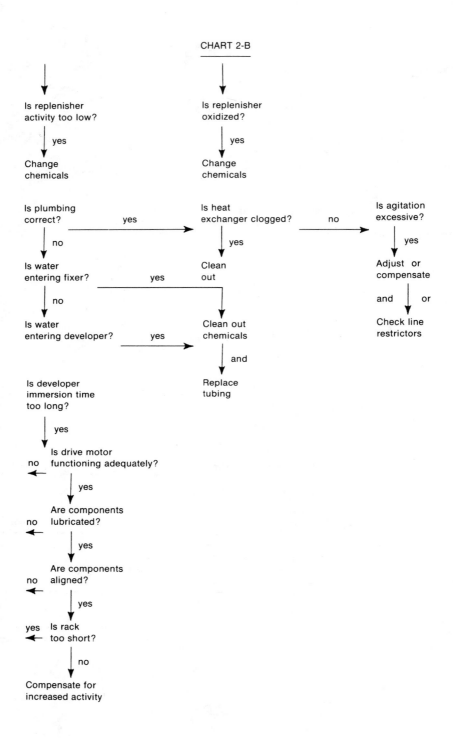

CHART 3-A

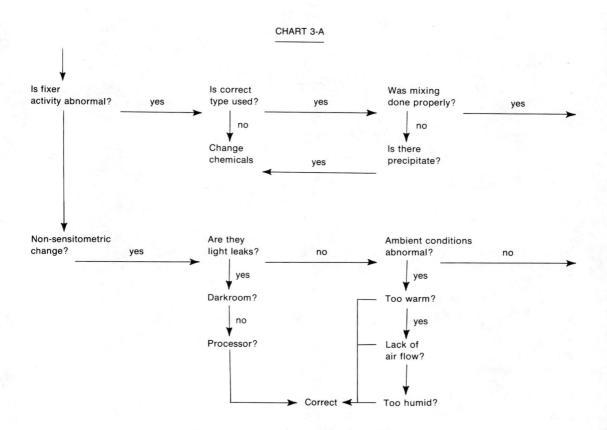

CHART 3-B

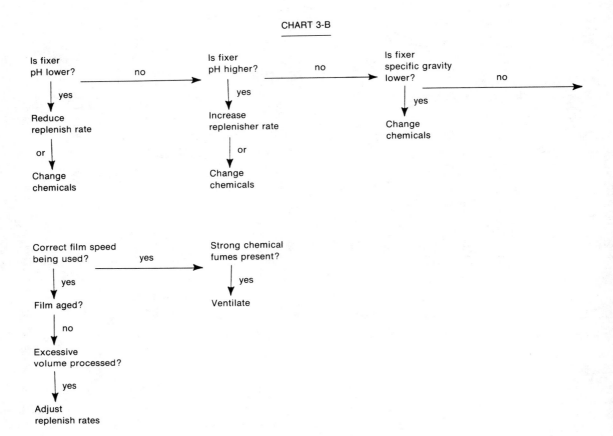

CHART 3-C

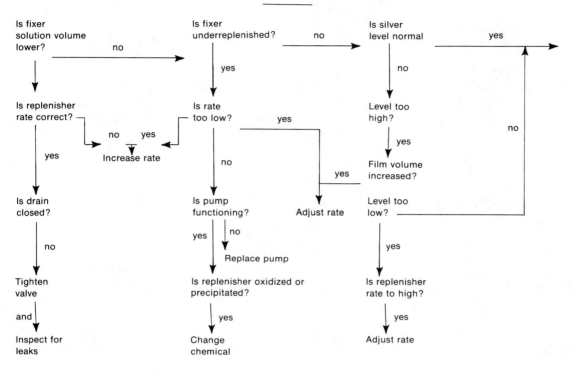

CHART 3-D

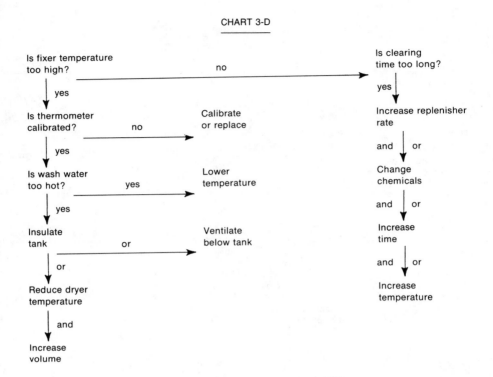

Chapter 9

Film Artifacts

Defined

An artifact is a defect in the film itself, although the word *defect* might refer to a medical problem seen in a film. An artifact is often thought of as something made by (human) hand. Radiographic artifacts may be made by humans, machines, or chemicals but are easily grouped as sensitometric or physical.

Sensitometric

Sensitometry deals with density levels and has four measurable values: maximum density (D_{max}), minimum density (D_{min}), speed, and contrast. These are the factors that govern the definition of image quality. An artifact is usually an increase or a decrease in density. If it is uniform increase in density overall, it is called fog (noninformational density) or an increase in speed. If there is a change in the density level in the toe or shoulder of the H & D curve, then there is a contrast change. Sensitometric changes could be due to any of the causes described in the paragraphs that follow.

Physical

Physical artifacts involve physical damage to the gelatin binder of the emulsion layer. Guide shoe scratches, roller pick-off, overdrying, and oil in chemicals or on the hands are examples (Fig. 9-1). Rough handling causes

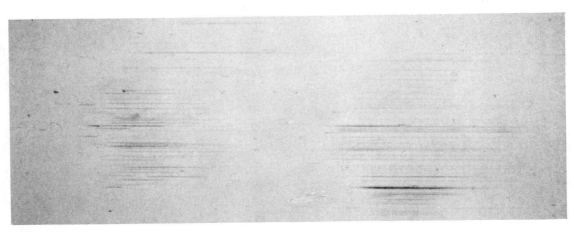

Fig. 9-1.   Fingertips pushed down on feed tray.

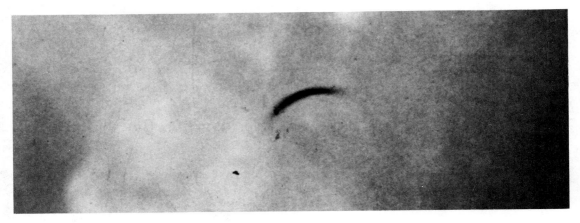

Fig. 9-2.   Sensitized kink mark.

kink marks (fingernail or crescent marks), physical damage that is seen as a mark that is simply a pile of silver or increased density with little or no indication of structural damage (Figs. 9-2 and 9-3). Physical damage is often expressed in terms of increased or decreased density also.

Sources

Darkroom/Handling

Radiographic film is a technological wonder, and one important element is that thousands of square meters (or feet) of film are made at one time. Many tests along the way weed out defective product. However, film that is less than perfect occasionally reaches the user. The manufacturer is usually

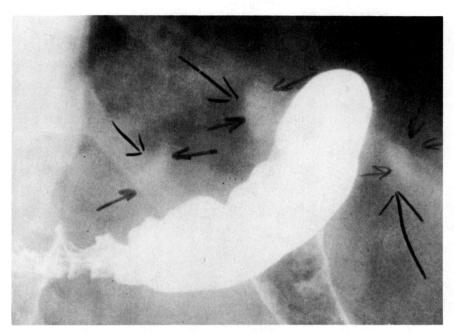

Fig. 9-3.   Desensitized kink marks.

less often the cause of a problem than are other factors, and there are tests that can be made to verify or refute this. If one emulsion number for a brand and type of film presents a problem, test another emulsion number. Next test the original box by selecting films from the front, middle, and back. Next feed films through the processor in two different directions. Each test, depending on the type of artifact, might be unexposed film, white light flashed, or sensitized by radiation to simulate a patient exposure. If one box is found to be unacceptable, set it aside and call the representative. Emulsion numbers are very important to artifact determination and for record keeping.

Before exposure, there could be variations in storage conditions, temperature, and humidity during the course of a day. Also, boxes of film should always be stored on edge to prevent pressure marks and damage due to accidental bumping.

After exposure, a film is two to five times more sensitive and will pick up artifacts more easily in this condition. This is why an artifact often appears on a patient film but not on a clear (unexposed) sheet that is processed. Any basic tabletop exposure of about 70 kVp and 2 to 10 mAs at 100 cm (40 inches) to produce a density of about 0.50 will be sufficient.

After processing, the influence of the view box and viewing ambient conditions affect the interpretation of film. Light is measured in foot-candles (lumens per square meter). A light meter set at ASA 100 and reading directly from a view box should read an exposure value (EV) of 13, which translates into 500 foot-candles. An EV of 12 represents a 50% reduction of light to 250 foot-candles, so all films appear darker than they are. A level of EV 14 represents twice the light at 1000 foot-candles, so all films appear too light. Films are often reviewed, checked, and sorted in ambient (background) light conditions of EV 10, whereas the radiologist reads the film in light of EV 4 to 6. With lower background light, the pupils of the eyes open and more information will be seen in the film. Under bright conditions, less is seen. All view boxes are a major source of contrast deficiencies seen in radiographs. When one bulb goes bad in a view box, replace all bulbs to ensure uniform color and light.

Exposure

Over- and underexposure, motion, distortion, geometric unsharpness, penumbra, and umbra all are well understood by the technologist. There are about 20 factors that contribute to latent image formation. In processing, there are only three components (time, temperature, and activity) controlled by seven systems. The chance of an artifact being produced by exposure inequities is greater in a controlled department. In an institution lacking processor quality control, the processor may be found to produce more artifacts simply because exposures are more closely controlled. However, it is important not to dismiss an artifact on a film as obviously being produced by darkroom/handling or processing. There are just too many exposure variables, and, despite the very best of controls, patients themselves must surely introduce a set of variables. One valuable clue in evaluating fogged findings is to inspect the nonscreen area at the edge of the film. If it is fogged, then age or processing is suspect. If it is clear and yet the film is too dark, then overexposure is the cause.

Processing

The electromechanical device and the chemical reaction in processing can alter the film in a variety of ways, from underdevelopment to overdevelopment, overswollen films resulting in wet pressure sensitization, or emulsion pick-off. The film might be scratched, resulting in plus or minus density depending on whether it occurred prior to fixation or after fixation. The film might be unclear, unwashed, wet, or dirty, or it may jam or slip in transport. All of the above problems can be caused by a variety of factors. One factor, the quality of the developer hardener, could cause most of these problems. Chemical failure will often be the cause rather than mechanical failure, because processing is a chemical system.

Clues

Film Stencil

Various manufacturers stamp an identification name or abbreviation on the edge of the film (Fig. 9-4). Some use a code to indicate type of film or batch, etc. One company prints the entire emulsion number on the film, and this is most useful for record keeping and troubleshooting. When confronted with an artifact, look for the stencil to verify film brand and type. The stencil is usually cut into the emulsion layer so that if it is lost in a high-density area the impression can still be seen.

Screen Stencil

Screen stencil is printed on the screen, so it blocks light from reaching the film and appears white (Fig. 9-5). Various manufacturers print their name and/or product name and/or emulsion or batch number. With greater emphasis on faster screen systems, it is important always to check the screen identification. It might be found that one set of older, slower screens was not changed, causing lighter film using current techniques.

Patient Identification

Almost every quality control technologist, chief technologist, or instructor has been presented with an artifact film and has sought the cause in the processor, darkroom, etc., only to find that they are looking at a patient's file film that is a month or 5 years old. Always look at the identification for the date and time. Next note the patient's age. If the film has not been used with

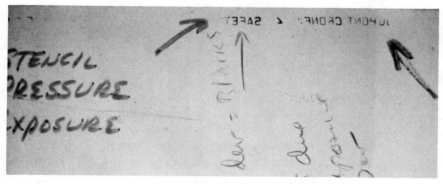

Fig. 9-4.   Film stencil.

Fig. 9-5.   Screen stencil.

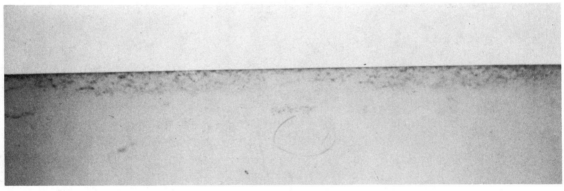

Fig. 9-6.   Wet pressure sensitization repeating pattern.

a patient and yet you can see the outline of the lead blocker area, this means the film was exposed in a cassette.

Direction of Travel

Look around the film edges for guide shoe finger marks, which will be in the direction of travel or across the leading and trailing edges (Fig. 9-6). Usually but not always, the more uniform patterns will be on the leading edge. The measured spacing of fingers will provide a clue to which processor is involved. Run down (trailing edge) or run back (leading edge), which is generally called curtain effect and is chemical stain, will also indicate direction of travel. Bromide drag (depression of density in the following area) indicates leading edge and direction. Wet pressure sensitization invariably is heavier on the outside edges as a result of greater roller pressure at their extremes. Gelatin strings or chevrons indicate direction of travel.

Repeating Patterns

The circumference of a roller is pi times the diameter. Pi is the mathematical constant 3.14. Thus the following chart may be constructed:

Roller diameter		Circumference	
Centimeters	*Inches*	*Centimeters*	*Inches*
1.27	.50	3.99	1.57
1.90	.75	5.97	2.36
2.54	1.00	7.98	3.14
3.81	1.50	11.96	4.71
5.08	2.00	15.95	6.28
7.62	3.00	23.93	9.42

Dirt or roller structural damage such as a gouge will repeat its pressure with every revolution (Fig. 9-7). When investigating artifacts with multiple

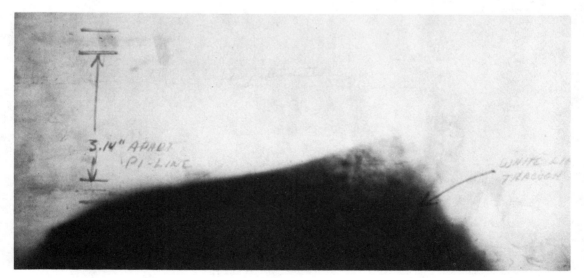

Fig. 9-7.   Repeating patterns: pi lines.

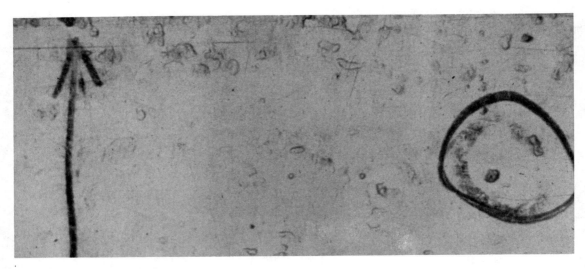

Fig. 9-8.   Wet pressure sensitization.

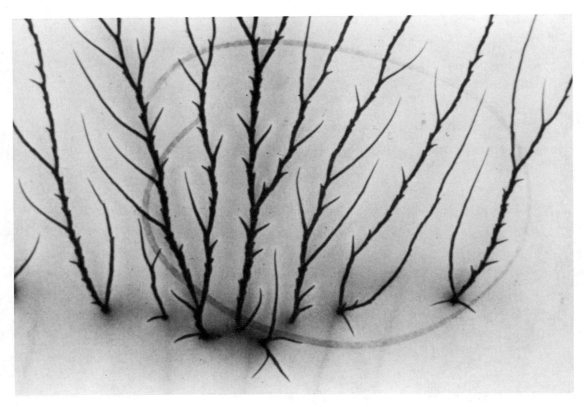

Fig. 9-9.   Tree static.

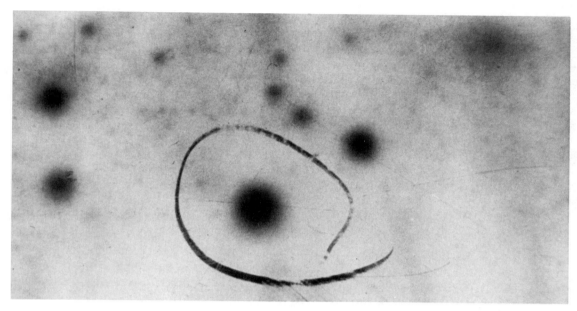

Fig. 9-10.   Smudge static.

points in the direction of travel, obtain a ruler and begin to look for repeating patterns. Remember that one roller might produce a variety of patterns, but most of them will repeat. These marks might be pick-off, wet pressure sensitization, edge crushing, chemical stain, oil spots, tree and smudge static shown in Figures 9-8, 9-9, and 9-10.

Viewing Conditions

Transmitted Light

A film is normally viewed in transmitted light. However, remember that the eyes are affected by the brightness of light, whether from the intensity of the light through the film, from other view boxes, or from room lights. Reduce the level of the ambient lighting and block off or turn off adjacent view boxes.

If the artifact is not seen or understood in transmitted light, remove the film and hold it about 10 cm (4 inches) from the view box. Based on the inverse square law, this reduces the light intensity. Angle the film left or right, top or bottom to provide further variations.

Reflected Light

Viewing in reflected light requires taking the film down and looking at its surface in the glare of the view box. Remember that there are two emulsions and both must be inspected.

Viewing in subdued light means removing the film from the view box, turning away from the view box, and looking at the film using light bouncing off the walls and ceiling. This method should provide the most amount of information. Check both film surfaces.

Bright Light

Bright light may help in seeing artifacts in very dark areas. However, most of these units work by a simple on/off switch or variable rheostat. In the first case, the light might be too bright and "burn through" the problem. In the second case, a radiologist might use one setting or intensity and a technologist another setting. It is difficult at best to use a bright light reliably for reading radiographs (good or artifact films).

Artifact Listing

With any artifact, try to categorize it as sensitometric or physical. Identify the general source (darkroom, exposure, processing) and check out all available clues. There are no perfect films, so concentrate only on the specific complaint but use all available clues including other artifacts of lesser importance than the primary one. A list of artifacts follows.

Low Density

I. Underexposure
   A. Wrong exposure factors
      1. Kilovoltage too low
      2. Milliamperage too low
      3. Exposure too short
      4. Focal-film distance too great
   B. Meters out of calibration
   C. Timer out of calibration
   D. Inaccurate settings of meter or timer
   E. Drop in incoming line voltage
      1. Elevators, welders, furnaces, blowers, etc. on same circuit
      2. Insufficient size of power line or transformers
   F. Photocell timer out of adjustment
   G. Incorrect centering of patient to photocell

H. Central ray of x-ray tube not directed on film; x-ray tube rotated in casing
    I. Distance out of grid radius
    J. Bucky timer inaccurate
    K. One or more valve tubes burned out (full-wave rectifying machines)
II. Underdevelopment
    A. Improper development
        1. Time too short
        2. Temperature too low (hydroquinone inactive below 13°C [55°F])
        3. Combination of both
        4. Inaccurate thermometer
    B. Exhausted developer
        1. Chemical activity used up
        2. Activity destroyed by contamination
    C. Diluted developer
        1. Water added to raise level instead of fresh developer
        2. Melted ice from cooling attempt
        3. Water overflowed from wash tank
        4. Insufficient chemical mixed originally
        5. Improper additions
    D. Incorrectly mixed developer
        1. Exact capacity of tank unknown
        2. Mixing ingredients in wrong sequence
        3. Omission of ingredients
        4. Unbalanced formula composition
        5. Overdose of sodium bicarbonate as retarder in concentrated developer during hot weather

High Density

I. Overexposure
    A. Wrong exposure factors
        1. Kilovoltage too high
        2. Milliamperage too high
        3. Exposure too long
        4. Focal-film distance too short
    B. Meters out of calibration
    C. Timer out of calibration
    D. Inaccurate setting of meters or timer
    E. Surge in incoming line voltage
    F. Photocell timer out of adjustment
    G. Incorrect centering of patient to photocell

II. Improper development
    A. Time too long
    B. Temperature too high
    C. Combination of both
    D. Inaccurate thermometer
    E. Insufficient dilution of concentrated developer
    F. Omission of bromide when mixing
III. Fog (see section on fog)
    A. Light-struck
    B. Radiation
    C. Chemical
    D. Film deterioration

Low Contrast

I. Overpenetration from too high kilovoltage
    A. Overmeasurement of part to be examined
    B. Incorrect estimate of material or tissue density
    C. Meters out of calibration
    D. Meters inaccurately set
    E. Surge in incoming line voltage
    F. Undermeasurement of focal-film distance
II. Scattered radiation
    A. Failure to use Bucky diaphragm
    B. Failure to use stationary grid
    C. Failure to use cutout diaphragm
    D. Failure to use suitable cones
    E. Failure to lead backing cassette
III. Exposure too short
    A. Timer out of calibration
    B. Timer inaccurately set
    C. Overload relay kicked out
IV. Improper development

High Contrast

I. Underpenetration from too low kilovoltage
    A. Undermeasurement of part to be examined
    B. In parts of varying thickness, setting of kilovoltage for thinner sections
    C. Meters out of calibration
    D. Meters inaccurately set

E. Drop in incoming line voltage
  1. Elevators, welders, furnaces, etc. on same line
  2. Insufficient size of power line or transformer
F. Overmeasurement of focal-film distance
II. Exposure too long
  A. Timer out of calibration
  B. Timer inaccurately set
III. Improper development

Fog

I. Unsafe light
  A. Light leaks into processing room
    1. Leaks through doors, windows, etc.
    2. Poorly designed labyrinth entrance
      a. Bright light at outer entrance
      b. Reflection from white uniforms of persons passing through
    3. Sparking of motors
      a. Ventilating fans
      b. Dryer fans
      c. Mixers such as for barium
    4. Light leaks in film-carrying box
  B. Safelights
    1. Bulb too bright
    2. Improper filter
      a. Not dense enough
      b. Cracked
      c. Bleached
      d. Shrunken
  C. Turning on light before fixation is complete
  D. Luminous clock and watch faces
  E. Lighting matches in darkroom
  F. When film is carried from machine to darkroom in containers, container may leak light
II. Radiation
  A. Insufficient protection
    1. During delivery or transportation in laboratory or shop
    2. Film storage bin
    3. Loaded cassette racks; steel back should face toward source of radiation
    4. Not enough protection for loading darkroom

B. Improper storage
  1. Radium
  2. Isotopes
  3. X-ray machines
III. Chemical
  A. Prolonged development
  B. Developer contaminated (foreign matter of any kind, e.g., metals, etc.)
IV. Deterioration of film
  A. Age (use oldest film first)
  B. Storage conditions
    1. Temperatures too high
      a. Hot room
      b. Cool room but near radiator or hot pipe
    2. Humidity too high
      a. Damp room
      b. Moist air
    3. Ammonia or other fumes present in darkroom or other working area
  C. Delivery conditions
    1. Moisture precipitation when cold box of film is opened in hot, humid room
    2. Fresh boxes should be stored overnight at room temperature before opening
V. Excessive pressure on emulsions of unprocessed film
  A. During storage
  B. During manipulation in darkroom
VI. Loaded cassettes stored near heat, sunlight, or radiation

Stains on Radiographs

I. Yellow
  A. Exhausted, oxidized developer
    1. Old
    2. Covers left off
    3. Scum on developer surface
      a. Oil from pipelines
      b. Impure water used when mixing
      c. Dust
  B. Prolonged development
  C. Insufficient rinsing
  D. Exhausted fixing bath

II. Dichroic
  A. Old, exhausted developer; colloidal metallic silver
  B. Nearly exhausted fixer
  C. Developer containing small amounts of fixer or scum
  D. Films partially fixed in weak fixer, exposed to light, and refixed
  E. Prolonged intermediate rinse in contaminated rinse water
III. Green tinted
  A. Prolonged immersion in chrome alum fixing bath
  B. Insufficient washing

Deposits on Radiographs

I. Metallic
  A. Oxidized products from developer
  B. Silver salts reacting with hydrogen sulfide in air to form silver sulfide
  C. Improper solder used in repair of hangers
  D. Silver-loaded fixer
II. White or crystalline
  A. Milky fixer
    1. Acid portion added too fast while mixing
    2. Acid portion added when too hot
    3. Excessive acidity
    4. Glacial acetic acid mistaken for 28%
    5. Developer splashed into fixer
    6. Insufficient rinsing
  B. Prolonged washing
III. Grit
  A. Dirty water
  B. Dirt in dryer

Marks on Emulsion Surfaces

I. Runs
  A. Insufficient fixing
    1. Weakened fixer
    2. Unbalanced formula
    3. Exhausted ingredients
    4. Low acid content
      a. Deficient when fresh
      b. Diluted from rinse water
      c. Neutralized by developer because of insufficient or no rinsing

    B. Drying temperature too high

    C. Contact with hot view box

  II. Blisters (formation of gas bubbles in gelatin)

    A. Carbonate of developer reacting with acid of fixer

    B. Unbalanced processing temperatures

       a. Combination of hot fixer and cool developer

       b. Combination of cool fixer and hot developer

    C. Excessive acidity of fixer or stop bath

    D. No agitation of film when first placed in fixer

  III. Reticulation

    A. Nonuniform processing temperatures

      1. Developer (hot)

      2. Rinse

      3. Fixer (cool)

      4. Wash

    B. Weakened fixer with little hardening action

  IV. Frilling

    A. Weakened fixer with little hardening action

    B. Hot processing solutions

      1. Developer

      2. Rinse

      3. Fixer

      4. Wash

    C. Prolonged washing

  V. Air bells

    A. Air bubbles trapped on film surfaces preventing development

    B. Extremely low humidity

    C. Failure to use wetting agent

    D. Puddles (buckshot marks; drops of water striking semidried emulsion surface)

    E. Streaks (drops of water running down semidried emulsion surface)

      1. Water trapped on hanger frames

      2. Water splashes

      3. Dirty hangers

      4. Drying airflow too rapid

  VII. White spots

    A. Screens pitted

    B. Grit or dust present on film or screens

    C. Chemical dust settling on film or screens (particles of certain chemical dusts will also cause black spots)

  VIII. Artifacts

    A. Crescents—rough handling

    B. Smudge marks—fingerprints or finger abrasion

C. Bands in marginal areas usually due to screen-mounting medium

Slow Drying

I. Waterlogged films
   A. Insufficient hardening in fixer
      1. Fixing period too short
      2. Weakened fixer from splashing
      3. Exhausted fixer
      4. Insufficient acidity
   B. Prolonged washing
   C. Wash water too warm
II. Incoming air too humid
III. Incoming air too cold
IV. Air velocity too low

Brittleness of Finished Radiographs

I. Excessive drying temperature
II. Excessive drying time
III. Outlet air too dry
IV. Excessive hardening in fixer
   A. Excessive fixation
   B. Excessive acidity

Streaks on Radiographs

I. Insufficient agitation while processing
II. Fog
III. Chemically active deposits (dried Chemicals on hangers)
IV. Pressure fog
V. Scratches
   A. Careless handling
   B. Grit present in air, cassettes, or on illuminator
VI. Exposure to white light during fixing
VII. Uneven drying due to high temperature and low humidity

Lack of Detail or Fuzziness

I. Motion (tube, film, subject)
   A. Inadequate immobilization
   B. Exposure too long
   C. Vibration of floor

    D. Slipping of subject on mount

    E. Stepping on and off operator's platform during exposure where control and tube are mounted on common mobile base

    F. Failure to arrest tube vibration after positioning before making exposure

II. Poor contact of intensifying screens

III. Improper distance relationship

    A. Object-film distance too great

    B. Target-film distance too short

IV. Improper focal spot

    A. Too large

    B. Damaged (cracked or pitted)

Static

I. Low humidity

II. Insulation

    A. Use of rubber gloves, shoes, finger cots, etc.

    B. Insulated flooring

III. Improper handling in

    A. Removal from box

    B. Removal from interleaving paper

    C. Loading cassette

    D. Unloading cassette

    E. Loading hanger

    F. Films stacked before processing

Decreased Density

I. Underreplenishment

II. Developer temperature low

III. Exhausted developer. Drain and clean tanks every 6 months or 50,000 films, whichever comes first

IV. Developer improperly mixed

Increased Density

I. Overreplenishment

II. Developer temperature high

III. Contamination of developer with fixer

IV. Developer improperly mixed

V. Light leaks in processor covered or in light seal where processor enters darkroom

Failure of Film to Transport

  I. Chemicals improperly mixed
  II. Chemicals contaminated or diluted
  III. Chemical temperature too high
  IV. Incorrect replenishment rates
  V. Dirty racks, turnarounds, or crossovers
  VI. Racks or crossovers not seated properly or warped
  VII. Dirty wash water
  VIII. Overlapped films
  IX. Tacky films in dryer section
  X. Incorrect dryer temperature
  XI. Dryer air tubes incorrectly located or seated
  XII. Hesitation in drive assembly, causing film to pause in transit
  XIII. Film not tracking through the processor on a straight course

Scratches

  I. Guide shoe out of line or dirty
  II. Dryer air tube not seated properly

Processing Streaks

  I. Rollers and crossovers encrusted with chemical deposits
  II. Dirty wash water
  III. Film not hardened properly by chemicals

Drying Streaks

  I. Dirty air tubes
  II. Film not hardened properly by chemicals

Pi Lines (Thin black longitudinal lines running across the film [see Fig. 9-7])

  I. Deposits on rollers in the developer tank
  II. Most often produced by new machines and will usually disappear after 500 films have been processed

Insufficient Drying

  I. Temperature too low
  II. Dryer thermostatic control or heater inoperative
  III. High humidity in dryer section, indicating one of the following:
     A. Insufficient air venting resulting in back pressure

        B. Damper in exhaust line not open far enough
        C. Exhausting into an existing line carrying a higher pressure than that coming from the processor
        D. Lack of or insufficient air-conditioning
    IV. Film not hardened properly by chemicals
    V. Solutions too hot

Artifact Chart

The following chart is spread over seven pages. The pages do not line up, but the arrows do. There are two sections: loss of density (pages 193–194) and increased density (pages 195–197). It is suggested that these pages be placed on poster board and affixed to the wall so the poster can be for ready reference and to promote staff awareness.

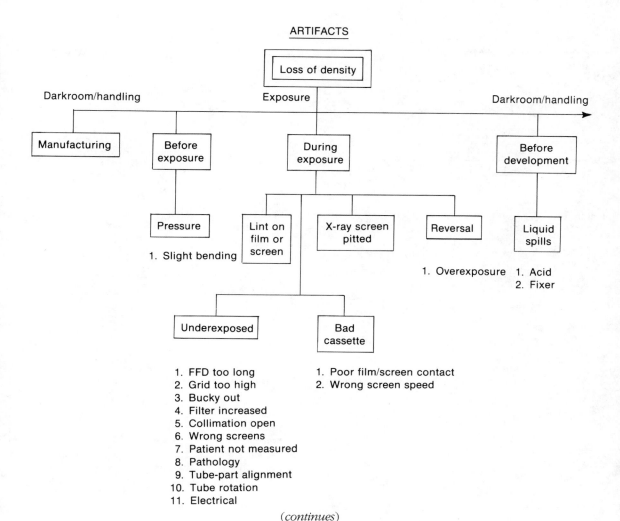

(*continues*)

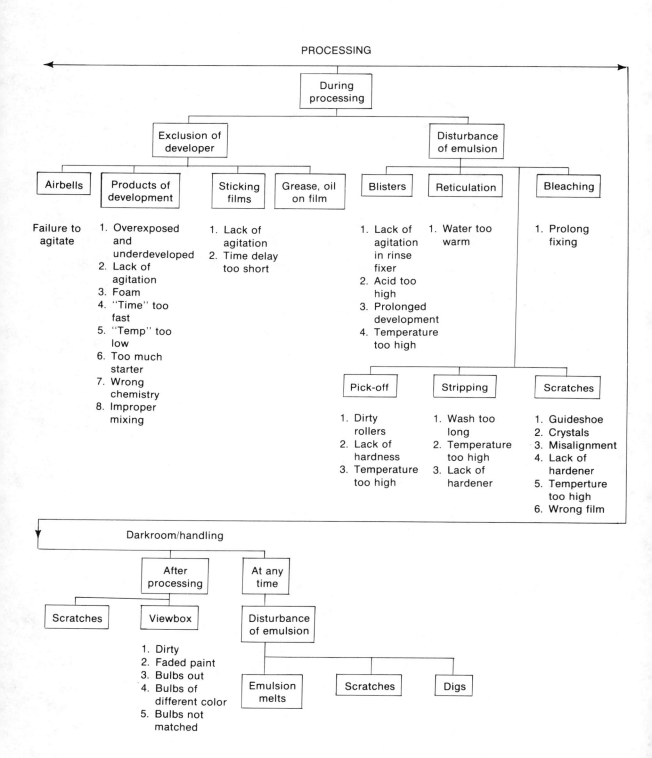

PROCESSING

During processing

Exclusion of developer

Disturbance of emulsion

Airbells

Failure to agitate

Products of development

1. Overexposed and underdeveloped
2. Lack of agitation
3. Foam
4. "Time" too fast
5. "Temp" too low
6. Too much starter
7. Wrong chemistry
8. Improper mixing

Sticking films

1. Lack of agitation
2. Time delay too short

Grease, oil on film

Blisters

1. Lack of agitation in rinse fixer
2. Acid too high
3. Prolonged development
4. Temperature too high

Reticulation

1. Water too warm

Bleaching

1. Prolong fixing

Pick-off

1. Dirty rollers
2. Lack of hardness
3. Temperature too high

Stripping

1. Wash too long
2. Temperature too high
3. Lack of hardener

Scratches

1. Guideshoe
2. Crystals
3. Misalignment
4. Lack of hardener
5. Temperture too high
6. Wrong film

Darkroom/handling

After processing

At any time

Scratches

Viewbox

1. Dirty
2. Faded paint
3. Bulbs out
4. Bulbs of different color
5. Bulbs not matched

Disturbance of emulsion

Emulsion melts

Scratches

Digs

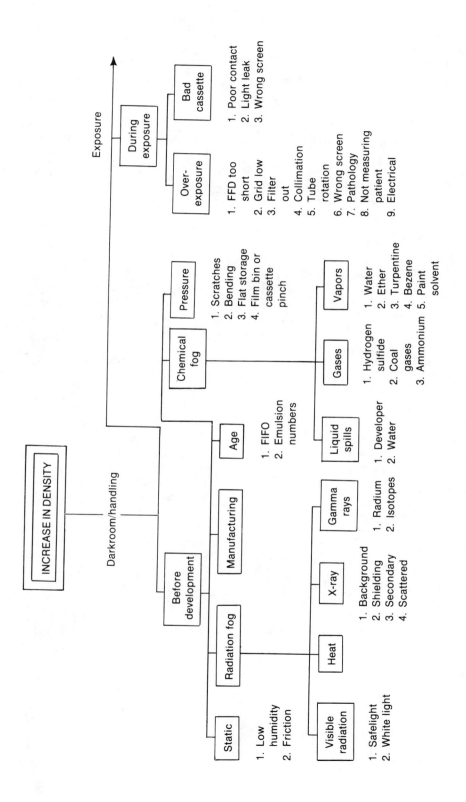

(*Flow chart continues*)

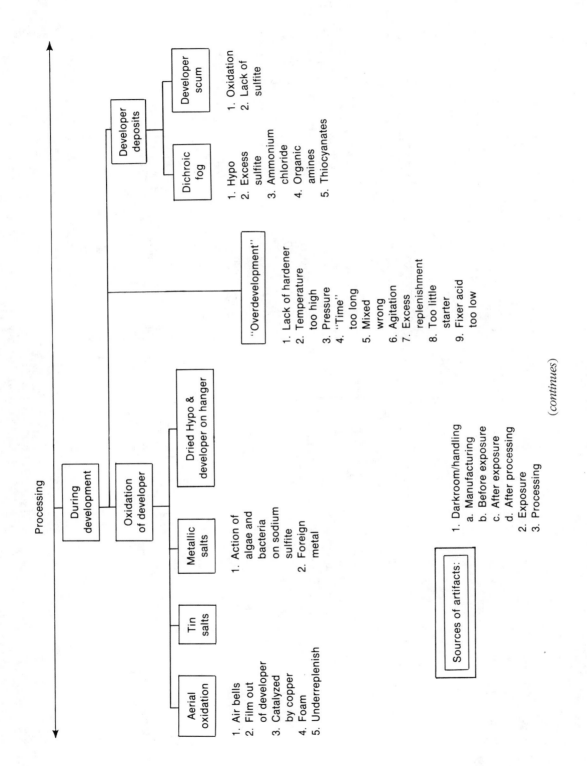

Processing

During development

Oxidation of developer

Aerial oxidation

1. Air bells
2. Film out of developer
3. Catalyzed by copper
4. Foam
5. Underreplenish

Tin salts

Metallic salts

1. Action of algae and bacteria on sodium sulfite
2. Foreign metal

Dried Hypo & developer on hanger

"Overdevelopment"

1. Lack of hardener
2. Temperature too high
3. Pressure
4. "Time" too long
5. Mixed wrong
6. Agitation
7. Excess replenishment
8. Too little starter
9. Fixer acid too low

Developer deposits

Dichroic fog

1. Hypo
2. Excess sulfite
3. Ammonium chloride
4. Organic amines
5. Thiocyanates

Developer scum

1. Oxidation
2. Lack of sulfite

Sources of artifacts:

1. Darkroom/handling
   a. Manufacturing
   b. Before exposure
   c. After processing
   d. After processing
2. Exposure
3. Processing

(continues)

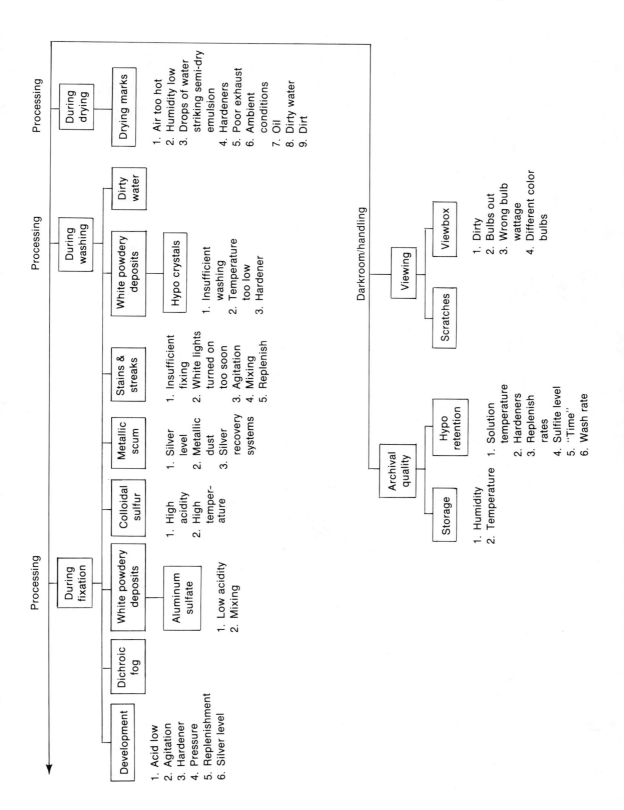

Chapter 10

Silver Recovery

Throughout most of the 1970s, silver prices were about $4.50 per troy ounce on the Spot Market for Industrial Bullion. In 1979, silver rose to $15.90 in September and amazed everyone by hitting almost $50.00 a troy ounce in January of 1980. Since then, the price has steadily fallen to below $10.00/troy ounce. Regardless of the price of silver, most institutions recognize the silver in the film as a recoverable expense. Most of the silver is recoverable. Unfortunately, it represents only about 10% of the purchase price of good "green" film, depending on the current silver prices and film prices. Thus much attention, some of it overstressed, is placed on silver recovery.

Reasons for Recovery

About 10% of the purchase price of film is recoverable. The exact amount depends on the film price, the silver price, the recovery efficiency, and overhead expenses such as service or refining fees. Any money recovered should be credited against a department's film budget, even if the money is returned to the institution's income pool. Another, and more technically accurate, method of determining the return on silver recovery is to consider the quantity of silver in a 500-sheet thrift pack of 35 × 43 cm (14 × 17 inch) or equivalent of green film. About 80% gross is recoverable but might range as high as 97% efficiency, but only 50% net can be reasonably realized in a very efficient department. This is because of expenses that will be discussed further on.

For environmental reasons, it is very important to remove dissolved silver from the fixer before fixer is passed to a sewer line, since silver in this form is highly toxic. The Water Control Act of 1972 banned the placing of toxic substances in public waterways or sewer systems. The Resources Conservation–Hazardous Waste Act of 1976 requires that available devices be used to remove toxic substances, and the clean water act* of 1984 requires the best available methods. The latest legislation is a federal law administered by the various states. The previous law was primarily a set of guidelines that were randomly enforced. The new law is called the Resource Conservation and Recovery Act (RCRA). It limits liquid waste to a toxic level of no more than 5 mg/L, which is the same as 5 ppm. Silver in used fixer or water is considered toxic. This level is approximately one-tenth that allowed in previous guidelines. Some municipalities such as Houston have levels that are approximately 10% of the new law.

The RCRA includes the requirement for permits to dump waste into public sewers for volumes greater than 27 gallons/month. This level is about 10% of the previous guideline. The public sewer is referred to as publicly owned treatment works (POTW). Discharge of toxic (silver in the fixer) substances to the ground, whether a septic system or open land, requires a permit from the National Pollutant Discharge Elimination System (NPDES) and/or the Environmental Protection Agency (EPA). If waste material is shipped to a refiner or treatment plant, a manifest is required: EPA form 8700-12 or form 8700-22. This includes silver recovery cartridges, flake, slurries, scrap film, and/or silver-laden fixer. Thus, considering the rather significant fines and sanctions for noncompliance, it is for environmental reasons that silver reclamation is practiced. If the system can pay for itself or make money, that is a plus factor to ease the burden.

Not much silver is being mined worldwide because of its low price and high refining charges. Photography uses the largest quantity and recovers about half of what is required annually. Obviously this represents a long-term losing balance.

Security

The silver recovery unit or scrap film must be protected against theft, and many departments have elaborate programs for these purposes. As noted above, one dollar's worth of green x-ray film contains about 10 cents' worth of silver. It should be obvious that very strict, or more strict, controls are

---

* This act was begun in 1984 and was vetoed in 1986 by President Reagan. Congress overturned the veto in 1987.

needed to protect the 90% part of the investment rather than the 10% of the investment. The economics become even more lopsided when one considers the expense of exposing and processing a film only to find that it must be repeated because of poor storage conditions. This is a counterproductive event that is very expensive and reduces the return on investment (ROI) while doubling the exposure to the patient. Every department should have an inventory specialist to control film supplies. Ordering, inventory, storage, and security all are involved. Monthly or even daily, films are accounted for to see if what was ordered was delivered and to see if the scrap plus exams equals the quantity used. A log should be kept of film delivered and when it is used. Emulsion numbers are very useful tools for keeping records. All film not in a film bin should be locked up. Film bins should be the type that prevents opening if any white light is present in the darkroom. Wasting an expensive box of film is the least expensive component compared with the other expenses involved in making a radiograph or the trauma, inconvenience, or hazardous radiation suffered by the patient.

Monetary Potentials

Green film represents an investment of about $2.00 per 35 × 43 cm (14 × 17 inches). Two 25 × 30-cm (10 × 12-inch), or three 20 × 25-cm (8 × 10 inch) films approximate one 35 × 43-cm (14 × 17-inch) film. Five hundred films (35 × 43 [14 × 17]) weigh about 18.14 kg (40 pounds) and contain 10 to 20 troy ounces of silver. Assuming the lower value of 10 troy ounces, that works out to 0.55 toz/kg (0.25 troy ounces/pound) of film. Of the total silver value, about 50% is dissolved into the fixer and 50% remains on the film. The silver in the fixer is carried out into the wash by the film at about a 5% level. Silver reclamation can do no better than 97% recovery of the silver and after expenses represents 80 to 90% recovery value. Thus, of the original 10 troy ounces, 5 went to the fixer and 80% equals 4 troy ounces recovered value. Of the silver on the film, another 5 troy ounces per 500 sheets of 40 pounds is about 100% recoverable, but the expenses are high so that only 30% silver value or 1.5 troy ounces is recovered. Thus, of the original 10 troy ounces 5.5 troy ounces are recovered net, or 55%. If the original 500-sheet box of film cost $1000, the green film silver value would be $100 ($10/troy ounces × 10 troy ounces). Net recovery of 5.5 troy ounces would return $55 ($10/troy ounces) or 55% of the silver value but only 5.5% of the green film price. Certainly some institutions can improve on these factors and increase their return somewhat. Any department should be able to obtain these basic levels. In any event, more silver (or more money) than what was originally designed into the products cannot be gotten out.

Processed film will vary in density and size, but one exhaustive study by the Du Pont Company using actual films purchased from a large medical center and the company's computer data bank on exam distribution and film utilization (cost analysis program) showed that 50% of the silver remains on an average film. An average film for a general diagnostic department would be about 30 × 30 cm (12 × 12 inches) or 900 cm² (144 m²), with an optical density (OD) level less than 2.00. A pediatric department or a chest changer would produce a different film size average and a different density level average.

Patient value is measured in the best possible diagnostic-quality radiograph at the least amount of radiation. The cost of the procedure becomes a secondary consideration. No amount of reclaimed monies can justify high repeat rates, which are hazardous to the patient and are economically unsound. This suggests that silver recovery practices must first consider the patient and film quality. Silver recovery units must not interfere with the processing of the film. Of course, a well-run department with effective quality control practices should be able to provide competent patient care and reduced cost through efficient silver reclamation. This does not diminish the legal or ecological need to recover silver to prevent pollution.

Silver Recovery from Fixer

Systems

Metallic displacement is also called metallic replacement, since a less noble metal such as iron in steel wool or screen is broken down in the acid fixer and displaced or replaced by silver atoms. Actually, the iron oxidizes, giving off electrons, which are used by the silver ions to form metallic silver. Recovery units of this type are called buckets or cartridges (Fig. 10-1).

Electrolytic units pass electricity through the fixer solution from a cathode to an anode. Electrons eroded away are used by the silver ions to plate on the cathode. These units are called cells.

Chemical precipitation involves a chemical that breaks down in the acid fixer, releasing electrons for the silver to use. The metallic silver is heavy, so it falls to the bottom of the container.

Resin systems are relatively new and are not yet commercial. They treat the resin particles with an acid to give them an ionic charge. Silver is attracted to the resin and picks up the electrons needed to form metallic silver. The resin must be retreated to remove the silver and recharge the column.

Methods

Centralized units are the single most efficient system, requiring the least amount of capital expense. The used silver-laden fixer is drained, pumped, or carried to a holding tank that feeds an electrolytic silver recovery unit. A single unit or cell will handle at least five processors because it is operating

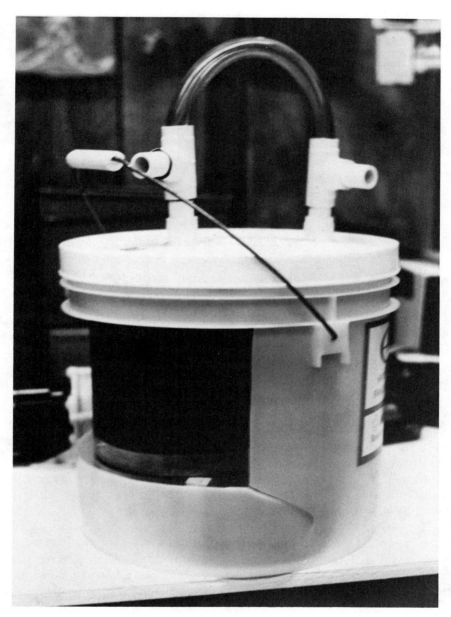

Fig. 10-1.   Metallic displacement cartridge with side cut open.

24 hours a day. It will operate at maximum efficiency, since the silver concentration is consistent and the flow is consistent from the holding tank. The holding tank of 114 to 190 L (30 to 50 gallons), stand, fittings, and tubing cost less than $500. Placing one cell at each processor would cost about $1000 per cell.

Decentralized recovery is the more common and expensive method of placing a recovery cartridge or cell at each processor. If the primary unit is inefficient, then secondary (terminal or tailing) units are installed. This consumes valuable floor space, increases fume production, and increases labor costs. The important consideration is to carefully size the recovery unit to the needs of each processor.

Percentage systems are a method of payment by an outside silver service (solution service, dealer). The service company provides the equipment and maintenance. About once a month, the silver is weighed and payment is made on an 80/20% split (approximately), with the larger portion going to the hospital. The department has no capital expense.

Silver services offer a plethora of deals, including the percentage mentioned above. Processor service and/or chemical discounts are often offered as inducements to allow the service to reclaim silver. Most of the inducements are offered as supposedly free or at a savings, but nothing is free. Compare the best prices for services and products against the value offered in the package deal. Next calculate the recovered silver value versus what is paid to the department under the proposed contract. In this way, it can be determined if a bargain is offered or not. Silver services might install their own equipment, buckets or cells, or collect the fixer and carry it back to their warehouse for recovery. The new pollution/recovery act of 1986 specifies that a license is required to ship silver-laden fixer to an outside service.

Selling used fixer seems curious, since the fixer has performed its job of clearing the film. What is cleared is the silver halide crystals, and this puts silver into solution at a rate of about 5.2 g/L or 6 troy ounces/gallon. If 10 gallons of used fixer containing silver at 0.6 troy ounce/gallon are sold at $5/troy ounce, that totals $30.00, or $3.00/gallon, which is probably greater than its original purchase price.

Factors Affecting Efficient Recovery

The fixer must remain within the recovery device for a certain period of time (dwell time) in order for silver recovery to take place. Passing silver-laden fixer through a unit too rapidly will allow most of the silver to flush through a unit too rapidly and down the drain. Adding a secondary unit increases efficiency by increasing the dwell time. This is the single most important factor.

Agitation is very important because it helps distribute the electrons so that they may be more efficiently used by the silver ions. Agitation keeps the solution uniform. In electrolytic units, agitation has a direct bearing on recovery capacity. In metallic displacement, agitation is caused as the solution flows around the steel wool fibers.

Surface area helps control recovery rates. The larger the surface area, the more silver can be extracted. Steel wool offers a very large surface area.

In electrolytic units, the larger area allows higher amperage to be used and thus a larger capacity for recovery.

Edges act as electron guns, and silver will plate at edges where electrons are more easily released.

Current flow is limited by an aspect of Faraday's law, but the general rule is that only so much amperage (per unit time) can be put into a solution. Low current is in the range of 1 to 10 A, while high current runs 10 to 20 A. In other areas of photography, units run as high as 70 A. Low amperage produces a hard, cream-colored silver that looks very pure. High average produces a softer, dark gray silver that is said to be burned. The purity is nearly identical, and the higher amperage will ensure greater efficiency. However, all units should have controls that allow the amperage to be turned up during busy times and turned down during slow times, and the control must be used. Using current at any level when no silver is present will destroy the fixer's thiosulfate, resulting in a smelly, yellow-brown deposit of sulfur. This is called sulfurization and is to be avoided.

Temperature is of minor consideration, as is pH, since these remain somewhat consistent. If the temperature is over 35°C (95°F) or if the pH is above 5, efficiency will drop.

Maintenance is required regardless of the unit used. These units require daily inspection and/or adjustment to ensure optimal operation and to prevent clogging, which can back up into the processor and affect patient films. The carbon electrodes in electrolytic cells should be scrubbed monthly with a stiff brush. All silver in the bottom of the unit should be removed and saved. Motors and shafts should be cleaned and lubricated as indicated in the operation manual. Maintenance is the single most overlooked aspect of silver recovery.

Metallic Displacement Systems

A less noble metal breaks down (oxidizes), giving off electrons that are used by the silver ions to form stable metallic silver. The lesser metal may be zinc, copper, or usually iron or steel. The metal may be cut-up screen, wound screen, or fiber as in steel wool. Steel wool may be either fine or coarse. The metal is usually housed in a 5-gallon plastic bucket, but a variety of sizes are available (see Fig. 10-1). Silver-laden fixer enters and flows down through the steel fibers. Silverless fixer is forced up the center and out the drain. In a controlled-flow, slow-rate situation, the bucket (cartridge) can be very efficient. However, radiographic departments have busy and slack periods. A bucket can only handle a prescribed quantity (milliliters per minute) of silver-laden fixer. Also, it operates at about 100% efficiency for only the first quarter of its useful life, based on total gallons or total silver. The efficiency falls to about 25% for the remaining three-quarters. Thus, the bucket should be changed frequently. If the bucket is loaded with water or silverless fixer, it will oxidize and lose efficiency since no silver is present. Trickling a very low volume through a new unit will result in steel consumption at a fast and inefficient rate. Placing too large a volume in the unit will flush out ferrous (iron) particles, which can react with developer to form ferrous hydroxide, which is a white, sticky, crystalline substance that clings to drains and eventually clogs them.

Buckets do not require electricity and are not a capital expense, but the unit does represent a renewable expense and it does require maintenance. Buckets should be stockpiled and shipped annually in large units to reduce bucket costs. They must be shipped with the acid inside. Draining off the acid exposes the iron to air, and a reaction that produces heat takes place. The silver ion sludge attacks the refiners' crucible, so they must charge handling fees that often are three times the fees charged for flake.

Electrolytic

Electrolytic systems are based on electrolysis or electroplating. An electrical current is passed through a solution between an anode and a cathode. The cathode gives off electrons that are used by the silver ions to become metallic silver. The silver clings or is plated on the cathode, which is usually made of stainless steel. These units are called cells because they resemble battery cells (voltaic cells) (Fig. 10-2). Each unit has a maximum recovery capacity in troy ounces per gallon, and this figure should be a guide in selecting the correct unit. To size a unit, determine the film volume in 35 × 43 cm (14 × 17 inches) for the two busiest hours of the two busiest days and find the average hourly rate. Next multiply by the replenishment rate, which is usually 90 to 100 ml/14 inches. This total is the number of liters (or gallons) per maximum average hour. Based on the silver content, the silver quantity per hour is defined and a cell of the next larger size would be purchased. A properly sized cell can recover 97% of the silver in the fixer. These are rotating anode, rotating cathode, or pump-agitated units. They may be terminal or recirculating, metered or batched, manual or automatic.

A single-terminal unit is usually the only requirement if it is properly sized. If undersized, silver will go down the drain, so a second unit is installed behind the first. The second unit is called a secondary terminal or tailing unit.

Recirculation units (Fig. 10-3) remove the silver-laden fixer, plate out most of the silver, and return the fixer to the processor. Since fixer is the least expensive component, a recirculation unit should not be purchased for the purpose of reducing fixer expense, which it may not do. Electrolysis destroys the sodium sulfite preservative, which in turn can lead to incomplete fixing and poor archival quality. To prevent this, the replenishment rate should be raised. Silver is never reduced to zero but must be maintained at about 10% of the normal level. The recirculation units usually have automatic

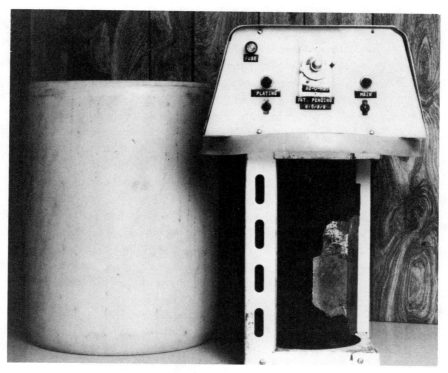

Fig. 10-2.   Electrolyte cell: silver partially removed.

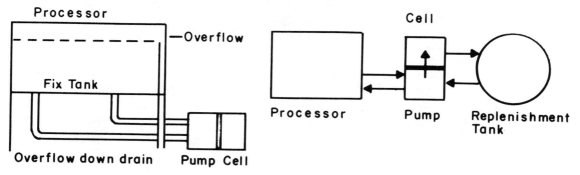

Fig. 10-3.   Recirculating silver recovery system.

controls and operate at low amperage. The main reason for using a recirculation unit is to meet specific environmental-pollution laws. The amount of silver carried out in the film into the wash normally is about 5% maximum, which is about 200 ppm and is further diluted by the water. However, the final silver content in the wash water may still be too high to meet local codes of 50 ppm. The recirculation unit keeps the silver concentration at about 10% of the normal level so that about 90% less silver enters the wash water, where it is safely diluted. Standard electrolytic cells can remove all but about 200 ppm, possibly requiring a terminal unit. A recirculation unit overflow is only 10% of the normal silver content of 0.6 troy ounces/gallon, or 0.06 troy ounces/gallon or 600 ppm. Obviously, another recovery cell is needed to capture this silver. Thus, recirculation units are expensive because of the autosensing-controlling feature, pumps, etc. They can serve a purpose in meeting a specific pollution codes but usually require another terminal unit. Recirculation units must have electrical and/or plumbing components connected to the processor. Even if the unit itself is approved by Underwriters Laboratories (UL) (or Canadian Standards Association [CSA]), it may violate the UL approval on the processor. It could also void fire insurance policies and local codes.

Manual control involves pushing a button or turning a knob manually to adjust the amperage and plating rate to the work volume at hand. In a typical 7 AM to 10 PM department, the level should be set at high until about 2 PM, assuming that 90% of the day's production occurs between 8 AM and 12 PM. The unit would be set at a midpoint from 2 to 4 PM and low for the rest of the period.

Semiautomatic units have on-off timers that turn the unit on in the morning and off at night. All units can have a timer added simply by using a retail security/lamp timer. These timers cost less than $10.00 and will handle 15A, while the largest recovery cell only uses about 5A because of built-in step-up transformers.

Automatic systems involve elaborate timer clocks, reference cells, and/ or computers. A reference cell is a miniature cell composed of an anode and cathode (Fig. 10-4). It monitors the relative ease with which electricity moves through the solution. A high silver concentration passes electricity easily in the unit, increasing the current supply. One unit adjusts the sensitivity of the reference unit to the specific gravity of the brand of fixer in use, since this will change the conductivity. Another unit is tied into the replenishment microswitch and monitors film feeding. As many films are fed, the plating current is increased; if no films are fed, the unit drops to its idle level. Automatic systems add considerably to the cost and must be checked daily to ensure that they are working. The reference cell must be cleaned monthly.

Precipitation

There are a variety of chemicals such as zinc chloride and sodium sulfite that will precipitate metallic silver. However, all of these are extremely hazardous, generating toxic (chlorine gas) and/or volatile (hydrogen) fumes. These cannot be used. One chemical precipitant that is safe is sodium borohydride. The Ventron Corporation division of Thiokol markets this chemical as Vensil. It is very inexpensive, works rapidly, but has two drawbacks. First, the pH of the fixer must be adjusted and tested several times a day. Second,

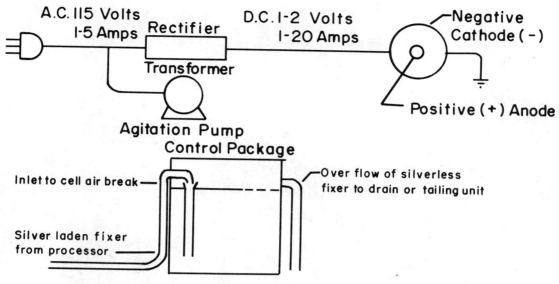

Fig. 10-4.   Electrolyte recovery.

precipitation would normally be done in a large drum, so either the precipitate has to be scooped out, dried, and packaged or means have to be available for moving and shipping the very heavy drum when it is filled. This method is very useful to dealers and may find its way into larger institutions, especially those with centralized recovery.

Estimating Silver Content

The amount of silver in a gallon of fixer or in a pound of scrap film has been discussed above. The important factor in determining a course of action or as a gauge of efficiency is to define the total quantity of silver in troy ounces and/or in dollar value. This then is the maximum, assuming perfect recovery, no loss, and no expenses. Since this is impossible, reduce the total to 50%. This is what should be accounted for at the end of a year. If the department meets or exceeds this level, it is doing an acceptable job. If it is below this level and there is no explanation, an investigation should be started to identify and correct problem areas. Silver value can only be recovered, and only half of the silver is in the fixer.

Testing For Silver Content

Silver estimating paper provides a reliable measurement (Fig. 10-5). Purchase a book of strips annually and keep it in a sealed glass jar away from fumes, moisture, heat, and light. The paper is used like pH test paper; however, the instructions vary with different brands. One company might instruct

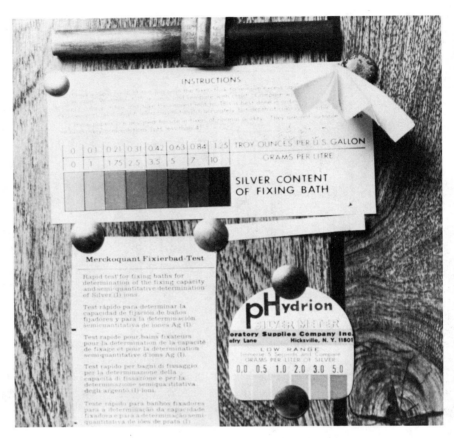

Fig. 10-5.   Silver test paper.

to immerse for 5 seconds, then read. Another company instructs to dip, wipe, wait 15 seconds, and then read. Follow these instructions exactly. Instructions will often state that reading must be in incandescent rather then fluorescent lighting. However, do not dip the paper strip and then try to find a lamp, unless this is included in the time period. The strip can become artificially darker with time. Also, the comparative reference patches are printed on bright white stock, so the test paper should be placed on an equally white surface. Test papers are most accurate in the midrange. If the silver concentration is above 0.6 troy ounces/gallon and reading is difficult, add an equal volume of fixer (which dilutes the silver concentration by 50%) and make a new reading, remembering to double the measurement. If the concentration is very low and it is difficult to decide if any silver is present, use a polished piece of copper (penny, pipe, wire, strip). Dip the copper in the solution and note the level of gray that is produced according to the following chart:

		Copper-Silver Testing	
Time (seconds) in fixer	*Amount of gray*	*Relative silver level*	*Troy ounces/gallon approximate level*
5	Dark, heavy	Very high	0.8–1.0
	Dark	Normal to high	0.6–0.8
	Gray	Normal	0.5–0.6
10	Light	Medium to normal	0.4–0.6
	Very light	Low	0.2–0.3
15	Gray	Medium	0.4–0.5
	Light	Low	0.2–0.3
	Very light, patina	Very low	0.1–0.2
	Clear	None	0

This obviously is a very subjective and yet a very sensitive test. It can be somewhat quantified by starting with a known high level of silver concentration and cutting this into low levels by adding fixer. After each use, reclean the copper with a scouring pad prior to the next test. The best time to use the copper test is during the busiest period of the day. Test the affluent from the recovery unit. There should be no silver leaking down the drain!

Maintenance

All silver recovery units require scheduled maintenance to be sure that they are clean and functioning properly. Most units are connected to the processor by a drain line. Fixer crystals can accumulate or grow inside this line, blocking it. When this happens, fixer spills over into the developer, causing ruined films. Spills over the side of the processor can cause damage to motors. Increased silver content in the fixer tank can damage the film (unclear, high hypo retention). These units must be checked daily and a record kept, even if the unit is owned and serviced by an outside service. Always be alert to electrical problems in cells because of the corrosive fixer and its fumes. Most electrolytic units lack UL approval for the simple reason that the electrical components are not isolated from the moisture and fumes. This poses an electrical problem (corrosion, inefficiency, error) and a hazard to people. Clean off the outside daily, look for leaks, verify the setting, make sure the electrical plug and tubing are connected, and record this activity in a record book. Whenever silver is removed from the cathode, clean out and weigh the silver in the bottom, scrub down the anodes, and remove all crystals. Never allow more than 2.54 cm (1 inch) of silver to accumulate on a cathode, or about half a kilogram (1 pound). Excessive thickness will short out or jam the unit, and excessive weight will burn out the drive motor in rotating cathode units.

Selling Silver

Flake is 90 to 95% pure when removed from a cathode of an electrolytic cell. It must be refined and assayed, and these costs are borne by the seller. The price for silver most often quoted is for the spot price for industrial bullion (99.95% pure) in the cash prices listing of precious metals of the *Wall Street Journal* (WSJ). Keep in mind that this is the selling price for finished product and not the purchase price for scrap. Thus, dealers who buy a department's scrap at the current WSJ price often deduct shipping, assay, refining, and profit from the quoted price. For example, there are 14.583 troy ounces per pound (avoirdupois), and a dealer might offer to pay 10 times the WSJ price of $7.00 per troy ounce. This means that the dealer pays $7.00 for each of the first 10 troy ounces and the remaining 4.583 troy ounces in the pound represents his expenses and profit. The important factor to note is that this amounts to about 30%, which is relatively high. Of course, instead of selling 1 pound, the department can stockpile and sell several pounds at once. The larger the volume, the lower will be the charges and the greater the multiplier. For example, a dealer might offer 12 times for 10 pounds and 13 times for 20 pounds. When selling flake, ask for bids from several refiners, bypassing the intermediaries. Sell once a year to reduce unit costs and to obtain the best price. When selling cartridges, stockpile and ship at one time to reduce expenses.

Silver From Film

Estimating silver value is discussed above, but the department should establish the total amount of silver available, the approximate silver per pound in green film, and the approximate amount per pound on black (processed) film.

Green film contains a quantity of silver from 10 to 20 troy ounces/500 sheets of 35 × 43 cm (14 × 17 inches). However, its weight is about the same as scrap or black film, which contains about 50% less silver. Since scrap film is sold on a per-pound basis, seldom is a price paid for green film that appreciates the silver content. Furthermore, film refining costs about two-thirds of the silver value. Thus, it is recommended that all green film be used for processor cleanup film. If for some reason a large quantity is involved, it is suggested that these be fed into fix, wash, and dry sections of the processor and then be discarded. The fixer will remove all of the silver that the recovery cell will adequately recover.

Black film usually means 5-year-old patient films from long-term storage but also includes scrap from current production, including repeats or cleanup film. It should include any film with density but not clear sheets. All paper and jackets should be removed. Sell once a year in the largest quantity possible after asking for several bids from salvage companies. Scrap green film is sold by the pound. The purchaser usually pays according to a figure based on the estimated silver content per pound. Most of the weight is the plastic film base, so the total weight is deceptive. In modern medical x-ray film, allowing that about 50% of the original silver is left on the film, there are about 0.10 troy ounces/0.45 kg (pound) of scrap or 10 troy ounces/45 kg (100 pounds). There are 12 troy ounces per troy pound, 14.582 troy ounces per U.S. (avoirdupois) pound, and 16 U.S. ounces per U.S. pound. In each case, the troy ounce is a unit of silver in a pound of silver. When discussing film, the discussion is the unit of silver weight (troy ounce) in a pound of film. Film weight is based on U.S. avoirdupois level.

Summary

Silver must not be lost down the drain because it pollutes the water, is in short supply, and represents monetary return to the department to help offset the cost of materials. There is only so much silver available for recovery, and after expenses only about 50% may be recovered by a department. It is worthwhile for the department to be as efficient as possible in silver reclamation, and this means daily involvement and checks. Keep very exact records of the photosensitive material (film) purchased and used according to type, size, and volume. Cross-check purchased silver value versus goal and actual return.

Chapter 11

Introduction to Quality Control

In radiography, a person makes subjective decisions when viewing a radiograph. The viewer might be the radiographer, processing technician, quality control supervisor, or photo interpreter (radiologist). A department tends to produce quality that is completely or partially dictated by the subjective preferences of the photo interpreter. Devices such as step wedges, penetrameters, sensitometers, and densitometers help to identify and quantify the quality level of production.

The final, visible image in a radiograph is a display of gray tones that relate to the exposed subject. Whether the scale of gray has the shape of a head or a casting or is simply a series of blocks, as in the case of a step wedge, they are all images. However, in the last case, the image quality can be more easily measured and analyzed. Sensitometry might be defined as the quantitative measure of the response of film to exposure and development. What this says is that one can measure quality if one controls the exposures and development of a piece of film. If several different films are given equal exposures and equal development, one may see and understand the different characteristics of the various samples of film. In a similar manner, for a given piece of film and a given exposure, development can be characterized. Exposure is similarly characterized. Thus, Hurter and Driffield provided a tool to measure or define quality. Remember, however, that the quality may be achieved by many variations and combinations of film, exposure, and processing. It is also influenced by the preferences of the individual for whom the films are prepared.

Once quality is somewhat defined by a radiographic department, how does one proceed to produce a uniform, reliable, consistent product (radiograph) time after time? How does a modern radiographic department issue the best possible results when presented with a subject of unknown quality? And how can the radiographic department best be operated, considering that it is a highly technical laboratory that is also a business? As a business, it functions like an assembly line to produce a high volume of consistent quality for the least amount of cost. A quality assurance program regulates quality, production, and maintenance. Quality assurance is an umbrella program that includes the tool more commonly called quality control.

The goal of quality control is to control quality, not necessarily to *improve* quality. Certainly, as better control is gained and observations are made, it may become obvious to the researcher how quality may be improved. However, that is not a defined goal of quality control. Because quality control is based on the quality of the controls, if poor controls, too few measurements, cheap equipment, or faulty records are employed, then the quality of this program and this tool will be reduced. Since quality control is a part of industry and the laboratory, we must look to these areas to find the best tools for implementing a radiographic quality control program. The best tool is statistics.

Modern radiographic quality control involves establishing a procedure for testing all of the components of the radiographic system: exposure devices, technique, film, holders, filters, processing, storage, viewing, etc. Usually, one form of testing will, by necessity, be used for the x-ray generator while another will be used for processing. However, statistical analysis would be the same for all data and should provide a unifying mechanism. Radiographic departments generally do not use statistical quality control and as a result have great difficulty in interpreting the data generated by their hard and sincere work. Statistics are confusing to many people and are a burden best left to someone else. Hopefully, this chapter will present just enough information to help some people better understand the basic concept of what quality control really means. Also, hopefully it will present just enough information to cause others to move to a higher level of sophistication in their quality control program. It is very unfortunate that everyone is not using statistical quality control methods and that they are often completely misunderstood. However, modern technological advances and economics dictate increased application of quality controls. Every manager knows that quality control is a vital economic tool and that it must have management support to succeed. The cost of producing a radiograph involves direct costs of equipment, personnel, and consumables, as well as indirect costs such as utilities, prevention, detection, and failure. The last three are a part of quality control.

If failure is measured as a repeat exposure expense of $10 to $20, it is easy to see that 100 to 1000 failures per year probably cost more than prevention and quality control. A simple evaluation of the return on investment (ROI) should convince most managers. Those still skeptical need only to analyze productivity levels when failure strikes. Most managers seek increased productivity as a way to reduce unit costs, but what manager wants increased productivity of poor quality or a low pass rate? Quality must be defined first and controlled second, and then productivity can be increased. Statistical quality control will provide information to aid in this process.

Finally, to the quality control supervisor goes the responsibility of control. This individual is not paid to be the resident technical expert who can solve problems, remedy mistakes, or correct failures, since these things only happen when there is a lack of control. The goal of this job is to prevent failures, mistakes, and a product that is out of control. Quality control charts, whether constructed traditionally or statistically, are extremely important aids to the supervisor. They provide past historical data, they indicate need for change, they indicate future failure, they document control, and mostly they aid economic-technological decision making.

Present Quality Control Procedures

Typically, a test is made and compared with a standard or against a specification. The test and the measurement are usually recorded. Generators might be tested twice a year, screens and film holders quarterly, and processing daily. These are, incidentally, all bare minimum test levels. In the case of more frequent processing tests, it is customary to generate quality control Charts. The test measurements are speed (speed point, speed index), contrast, base plus fog (B + F, net density), and perhaps developer temperature and background density. Speed and contrast are usually indicated values rather than calculated, since the latter can only come from drawing H & D curves. Besides, indicated values are adequate measurements.

For the speed indicator, a chart is constructed as in Figure 11-1. The midpoint is suggested by the film manufacturer, dealer, or some other source. Upper and lower limits are assigned based on the midpoint, usually at ±15%. These limits should indicate limits of acceptability. On day 1, a test is made and a measurement is produced (by "eyeballing" comparative analysis, or densitometer reading) and is posted on the chart. For example, let's say that the midpoint is 1.30 (Fig. 11-2). This really means a density reading of 1.30 for a controlled exposure on a controlled piece of film, hopefully processed through a controlled processor. Industrial radiography might have an aim point of 1.00 or 1.50 but usually 2.00, depending on the type of subject and other factors. On day 1, the densitometer reading of the control test strip

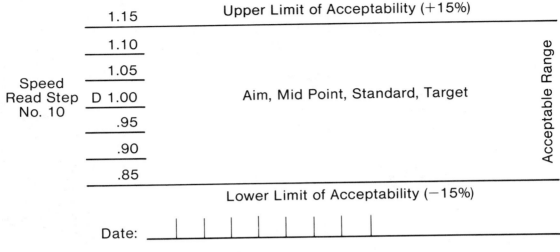

Fig. 11-1.   Trend chart for speed.

step (exposure level), which should produce a density of 1.30, produces a density of 1.40. What does this mean? Is it important? What must be done next? What is the cause? And, is it accurate (see Fig. 11-2)?

First, the reading may not be accurate, so recheck it. Also, make certain that the densitometer has been zeroed and that it matches the calibration point on its supplied reference test patch. Do this daily. Next, a midpoint is set ("aim" is a better word) at 1.30, but this is not an absolute value and is only a starting point. Perhaps after 10 to 20 tests it will be found that 1.24 is actually the true midpoint for this film, exposure, and processing used. If this is true, then the aim would be to the more accurate data, but this is discussed later. One test might measure 1.40—and that seems to be a problem—but remember, the chart was constructed with a ±15% limit of acceptability to allow for normal fluctuations due to uncontrollable variables. The chart states, "hit 1.30 if possible, 1.35 or 1.40 or 1.45, but do not go above 1.45 (plus 15% above 1.30)." Thus, there is nothing wrong with 1.40 as a reading, and there is too little information to make an inference about whether or not this is the beginning of an upward trend. Since ±15% is considered an acceptable variation, then the upper limit is the limit to acceptable quality beyond which there is unacceptable quality. This actually is not quite correct, because a film might still be acceptable if it were 20 or 25% too dark under certain circumstances. But there is a need to establish controls and to try to meet these goals if there is to be control. Initially, it is preferable to start with artificially large limits, and, after sufficient data are gathered and control instituted, the parameters (limits) may be and should be tightened. Returning to the example, it may be concluded that the 1.40 reading is of no particular concern. It is close to the midpoint and is within limits. It may also be deduced that only one test might represent random error, that one test really does not tell too much, and that a lot is riding on the interpretation of that one test. It is perhaps this last notion that most scares quality control personnel. They intuitively sense the nagging question, "Is this the beginning of a trend leading to disaster?" Therein lies the major defect in current quality control programs and trend charts: insufficient testing.

When the measurement of the day 2 film is plotted, it will be the same as day 1, greater or lower. Its position will add further information to day 1. Day 3 will provide still more information, and so on. Thus, the more information available, the easier the interpretation (Fig. 11-3).

If only one test is made daily, it might take a week to gather sufficient data upon which to base a judgment. Adding other measurements, such as contrast and B + F, yields additional clues that should help in interpreting what is happening. There is validity in responding to a preponderance of evidence. Imagine being able to have additional and more accurate data sooner. Testing at the same time each day will improve accuracy. Testing at least three times daily (7:00 AM, noon, 4:00 PM, or equivalent per shift) will generate increased data upon which to base judgments (Fig. 11-4). Even the wisest person has difficulty making decisions based on little information. Acquiring more information is always a wise move. Plotting only speed constitutes a single-point plot approach, which is better than nothing but is very difficult to understand. Testing only once a day is subject to the same criticism. Multiple testing with multiple points improves the data base, and the decision making is easier. Obviously, the reason for control charts is to aid in evaluating

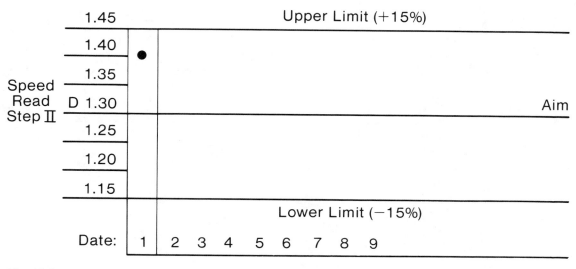

Fig. 11-2. Trend chart—speed.

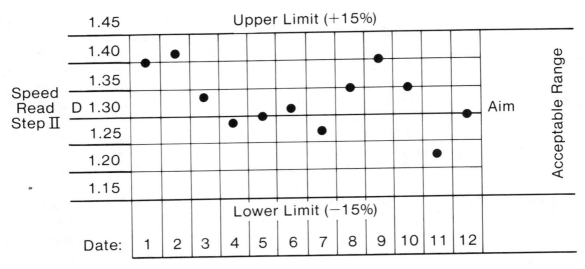

Fig. 11-3.   Trend chart: a picture of activity.

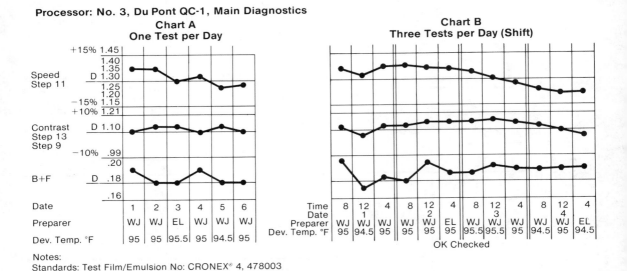

Fig. 11-4.   One test vs. three tests per day.

whether the process is in control, whether there is a trend out of control, and whether the source of error is a controllable or uncontrollable variable. Without making decisions based on interpreting the quality control charts, there cannot be control of quality. Interpretation is quite difficult for most people and is only practiced by a few.

The simplest interpretation begins when a test point is plotted on a trend chart beyond the limits of acceptability. Since it is outside the acceptable area, the interpretation is that something went wrong. One or more of the controlling factors is not in control. In radiographic processing, this could be the time (developer immersion time), temperature (developer temperature), or activity (developer chemical strength, bromide level, pH, specific gravity, agitation, and replenishment rate). These are controlled or controllable variables. Transport is usually stable to ±5% but may slow down to increase developer immersion time by 30% as a result of lack of lubrication or when roll film or only large-format film is fed in large quantity. There are, then, normal conditions and unusual or abnormal conditions. Temperature stability is controlled by the thermostat, the heating element, and heat exchangers to ± ½°F or better, usually. It can be relied on. However, the ambient temperature of the room or of the processor, water flow or temperature changes, film volume, dirt, and age all can affect accuracy of control, which directly affects overall film quality control. If the replenishment rate is incorrectly specified, then the chemical activity will change although the replenishment system is working correctly. However, if the correct replenishment is chosen but the work load changes, if the film type is changed, or if the electromechanical replenishment system fails, the chemical activity will change and will affect image quality. There are three gross areas that can be measured:

Electromechanics
Chemistry
Sensitometry

In actual practice, all three are monitored, and quality control charts (trend charts whether practical or statistical) may be constructed on the information gathered from testing. Since sensitometry is the sum total of film plus exposure plus processing (electromechanics and chemistry), it is chosen as the most universal test.

In summary, to understand better what is taking place in the radiography department, and especially in processing, trend charts are established for several different measurements (speed, contrast, B + F, etc.). Tests are made and the data recorded on the charts. The charts are analyzed to make certain that the system (processing) is in control. When the trend is toward out of control or is actually beyond the limit of acceptability, corrective action is taken to return the system to acceptable control. Unfortunately, all too many quality control people, who do have trend charts, use the practical rather than statistical methods and fail to interpret the data. For them the charts become simply a documentation of events.

Statistical Quality Control

Most people are immediately put off by the word *statistics*. They have heard that "you can prove anything with statistics" or that "it's very complicated math." Both are usually true. However, it is possible to understand a little about statistics and, as a result, make the job of quality control more productive and easier because of the heightened level of understanding (interpretive skills).

Statistics is the application of mathematics to problem solving and decision making. It can describe a large mass of data and/or be used to make inferences, predictions, and decisions. In making decisions, it finds application to the inherent goals of quality control: influential statistics. A trend chart represents a large quantity of data. If the speed point is tested and recorded on the chart over 20 or 30 days, trends can be seen within a week or within the month. This is the essence and purpose of the practical trend chart. In statistics, these data would be called a population—a set of data that characterize some phenomenon. The chart provides a graphic display that is easier to interpret than a row of numbers (numerical display). For a set of data, a relative frequency distribution or histogram may be constructed and some observations may be made. Most people call this a bell-shaped curve or gaussian distribution curve, which really indicates a normally distributed curve graph as opposed to a skewed or nonuniform one. Statistics expects to find in a set of data a normal distribution and has some mathematical tests to see if this is true. The center of the bell represents the center of the population and is called the central tendency, or middle value, or median. The median is simply the center of the group, the majority of the test data. Median may be calculated by taking all of the speed readings (or contrast or B + F) for 1 month and listing them from smallest to largest. If there is an even number of readings, average the two middle readings. If the total number is odd, there will be only one center number. This is the center of the data, the center of the population. Based on the tests, you have just found the median or midpoint for the control chart. Instead of guessing where the midpoint should be, we have found where it is. (Fig. 11-5).

As an example, let's consider the speed point readings for 23 days. As recorded, they were 1.36, 1.39, 1.41, 1.22, 1.24, 1.29, 1.26, 1.21, 1.16, 1.19, 1.16, 1.28, 1.22, 1.13, 1.15, 1.12, 1.19, 1.18, 1.18, 1.17, 1.08, 1.10, and 1.17. (These are density readings of the same step in test films). Arranged in order, they are 1.08, 1.10, 1.12, 1.13, 1.15, 1.16, 1.16, 1.17, 1.17, 1.18, 1.18, *1.19*, 1.19, 1.21, 1.22, 1.22, 1.24, 1.26, 1.28, 1.29, 1.36, 1.39, and 1.41.

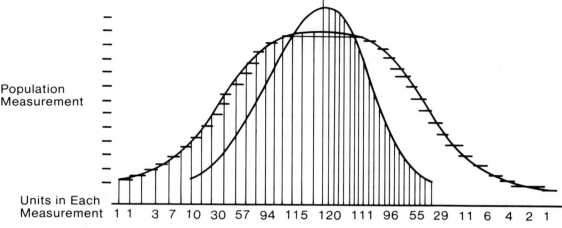

Population Measurement

Units in Each Measurement 1 1   3 7 10 30 57 94 115 120 111 96 55 29 11 6 4 2 1

Fig. 11-5.   Bell-shaped distribution curve.

The median is the position number 12, or 1.19; there are 11 readings below this value and 11 readings above this value.

Another measure is the average of all these tests. This is also expressed as the mean ($\overline{X}$, read "X-bar") of a set of quantitative data. It is calculated by finding the sum (Σ, or sigma) of the measurements (X) divided by the number of measurements (N):

$$\overline{X} = \frac{\Sigma X}{n}$$

In more sophisticated statistics, this is written as follows:

$$\overline{X} = \frac{\Sigma_{i=1}^{N} X_i}{n}$$

but is the same expression. Despite the unfamiliar symbols, what this means in basic, uncomplicated terms is simply that the average is found by adding up the 23 speed readings listed above and dividing by 23. In this example, the answer is 1.21. The average (or mean) is 1.21. This second piece of information may be added to the first to increase our understanding of what is happening. If there is normal distribution and the data form a perfect bell shape, the median and mean will be identical. In this example, the mean (average) is greater than the median. This means that the curve, or distribution, is not normal but is somewhat distorted. In fact, it means that the curve is skewed to the right. If the median were larger than the mean, the curve would be skewed to the left. Median shows central tendency (the center of the group); mean shows average but is influenced by extremes. A symmetrical bell (median = mean) is desired. When a curve is skewed, it indicates that there are a few extremes (high or low) that are pulling the mean to the left or right. It is important not to overact to a trend or data point based on a skewed chart. The skewed chart alerts us to the presence of extremes (Fig. 11-6).

Next this knowledge can be applied to analysis of entire trend charts (Fig. 11-7).

In Figure 11-8, the data are more wildly fluctuating, and there may be a weekly trend of a rise on the second and fifth day with a lower midweek. There is definitely a trend off the chart. However, the data are normally

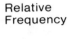
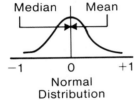
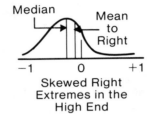
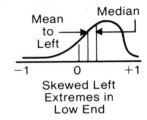

Fig. 11-6.   Mean and mode relationships.

Analysis of Trend Charts; Distribution of Data: Normal or Skewed

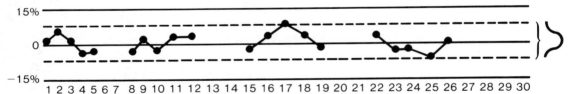

Fig. 11-7.   Distribution of data: normal/on aim. The data are close to the aim. There are no fixed patterns, no trends. The data for the month are normally distributed (bell-shaped curve). The mean and median are equal.

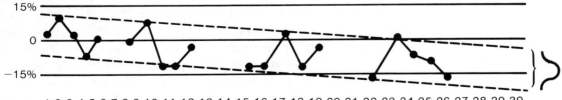

Fig. 11-8.   Distribution of data: normal/downward trend.

distributed for the month (bell-shaped curve), and the mean equals the median. This indicates that the entire process is changing rather than that one assignable cause is out of control. A skewed curve indicates a single cause and shows whether it is a high or low value.

But how does this relate to radiography? In Figure 11-9 are plotted the data from the example above. Note that data are plotted as read and that there are highs and lows. There are also weekly trends and a monthly trend. Are the data performing correctly, is the chart correctly constructed, and will it be interpreted correctly?

The obvious conclusion is there is a loss of speed over the month. The fact that the data are off the chart is interpreted as unacceptable, and the decision is made to do something about it—perhaps raise the temperature and/or the replenishment rate. Is this a valid interpretation? Yes, but perhaps it can be made more valid through statistical analysis. Although the chart has a speed point of 1.30, it has been learned that the median is 1.19 and the average is 1.21. These numbers are relatively close. If the speed point were stated at 1.20, there would certainly be better stability. Another measurement is the mode, which is simply the number that shows up most frequently in the data. In the sample above, there are two samples each, at 1.16, 1.17, 1.18, 1.19, and 1.22, so the mode indicates a very broad distribution curve with an arbitrary average of 1.18. This further suggests that this processor throughout this time period was relatively consistent and had a general fluctuation that was acceptable.

Returning to the discussion above regarding the skewed curve, where is the curve in the data above? (Fig. 11-10) The data are slightly skewed downward (to the right of center), and this indicates a general loss of speed over the month. Although this is an obvious interpretation without statistics, the magnitude of this error cannot be gauged without statistics (Fig. 11-11). For instance, below the data are drawn-in weekly segments with proper spacing. Below each weekly segment is the average (or mean) for the week. It can quickly be seen that the middle 3 weeks are very close, with a noticeably higher first week and noticeably lower last week. As you scan the numbers, you are probably thinking that the median is 1.19, the average is 1.21, but

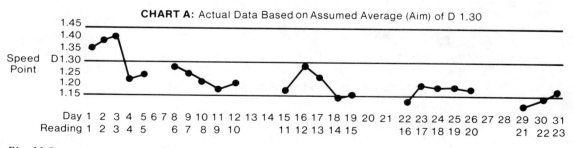

Fig. 11-9. Actual data.

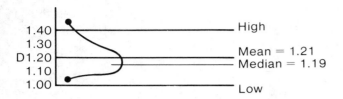
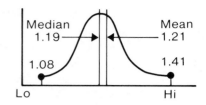

Readings: 23

Fig. 11-10.   Bell-shaped distribution curve of actual data. Extremes on these days have caused slight skew to the right. The curve on the left is redrawn on the right in the normal position.

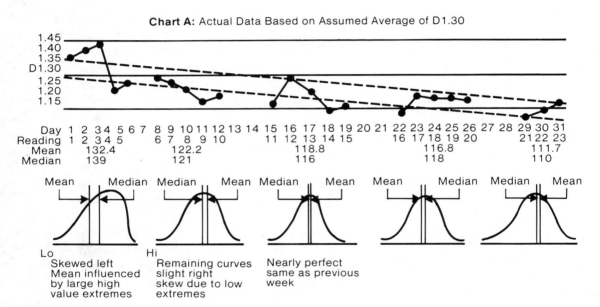

Fig. 11-11.   Actual data with weekly distribution curves.

the first week is averaging 1.32 and the last week is averaging 1.12. This explains the mode.

   Once it is determined that there is a more or less normal distribution of samples about the mean, it is useful to determine the variances about mean or how much the samples deviate away from the mean or central tendency. The sample standard deviation (σ) is the positive square root of the sample variance (σ^2), which is the sum (Σ) of the samples (X) minus the mean ($\overline{X}$) squared and divided by the number of samples less 1 (n -1), which is the degree of freedom (Fig. 11-12).

   Recalling that the mean ($\overline{X}$) was found to be 1.21, if σ (0.09) is added to it, a single deviation or one standard deviation from the mean is found to be 1.30 ($\overline{X} + \sigma$). Subtracting σ from $\overline{X}$ provides one standard deviation down

$$s = \sqrt{s^2} = \frac{\sqrt{\Sigma\,(x - \bar{x})^2}}{n - 1}$$

$$s^2 = \frac{\Sigma\,(x - \bar{x})^2}{n - 1} = \frac{\Sigma\,x^2 - \dfrac{(\Sigma\,x)^2}{n}}{n - 1}$$

$$= \frac{33.9146 - \dfrac{776.1796}{23}}{22}$$

$$= 33.9146 - 33.7469$$

$$= 0.0076$$

$$s^2 = 0.0076$$
$$s = \sqrt{s^2} = \sqrt{0.0076} = 0.087 = 0.09$$

Fig. 11-12. A sample standard deviation calculation.

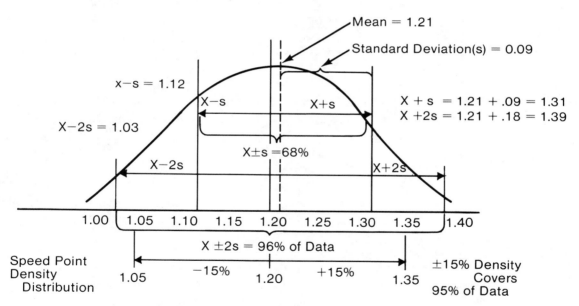

Fig. 11-13. Bell-shaped distribution curve: standard deviation limits.

scale ($\bar{X} - \sigma$) of 1.12. Analyzing the data should show that 68% of the 23 readings lie in this range. Similarly, 96% of the data points will lie within $\bar{X} + 2\sigma$* and $\bar{X} - 2\sigma$* or 1.39 and 1.03. Of all data, 100% should lie within 3σ variances (this is 3 standard deviations or 3 sigma variance) (Fig. 11-13).

* "σ" is lower case sigma (Σ) and is standard deviation (SD). In this example, $\bar{X} \pm 2\sigma$ is expressed as "± 2 sigma, standard deviation."

In radiography, the general rule is that the speed point limits of acceptability are ±15% of the speed point. In this example, that would range from 1.36 to 1.06, which is very close to the 2σ level (two standard deviations plus and minus or two sigma). Thus, it appears that this set of data has nearly normal distribution in a bell-shaped curve with a mean of 1.21. This is a stable processor at an average speed of 1.21 and not 1.30, as the chart is labeled. It could be very possible that this processor is underdeveloping, but that is not a concern. The concern is whether or not it is consistent and in reasonable control. With 95% of all data falling within the ±15% limitation, it is indeed in control. This might be better appreciated if the original data are recharted using a speed point aim of D (density) 1.20 (Fig. 11-14).

Shewhart Charts

In 1924, Walter A. Shewhart, of Bell Telephone Laboratories, found a way to graph running records of performance to see more easily if the process was in control and to facilitate making decisions. There usually are two charts used for each measurement: $\overline{X}$ (mean), which shows the process level with high and low peaks being undesirable, and R (variance), which shows the range of process variability, and only high points are objectionable. These together are called $\overline{X}$, R (read X-bar-R) charts. The $\overline{X}$ is simply the aim based on the average. The R is the range from the lowest to highest value.

Previously, there was mention of controllable and uncontrollable variables. Variability is a fact of life and, when it exists, does not mean it is unacceptable or that the whole system is out of control. When factors such as time, temperature, and chemical activity are controlled as much as is humanly possible, variation is reduced (quality is under control) but not eliminated. Chance or random events can cause process variability. Because of this, it is important not to waste time fixing something that is really acceptable or not taking appropriate action when indicated. Often, taking action is only

Chart B: Data Displayed with Found Median/Mean of D1.20

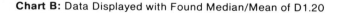
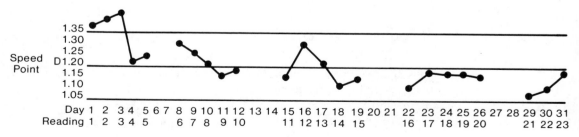

Fig. 11-14.   Data redrawn about found aim.

a learning experience because one cannot solve the problem (unassignable cause) or because it need not be solved or even adjusted. Many people who lack skill in interpreting charts make both errors, with the resulting confusion and frustration of technicians and management.

The purpose of control charts is to establish limits and to allow the analysis of data gathered. The basis of all control charts is the sample or date value (X), mean or average used as the aim ($\overline{X}$), range or variance (R), and standard deviation (σ). A properly constructed Shewhart $\overline{X}$ chart covers the midpoint or aim (really the mean or average based on previous testing) and $\pm 2\sigma$ of normal variability. Any point outside of the normal area is probably due to some assignable cause, such as developer temperature too high, overreplenishment, or transport slowdown. Shewhart believed that the process would dictate the limits about normal variation. This is how a true $\overline{X}$ chart is set up. Compare Figure 11-16 with Figure 11-9 (practical trend charts). The major difference is that the $\overline{X}$ chart is composed of at least five tests or samples per day or test period. The center line, midpoint, or aim is the mean. The upper control limit (UCL) and lower control limit (LCL) are ± 2 or 3 σ from the mean. This is also written as follows:

$$\text{Center line}_{\overline{X}} = \zeta_{\overline{X}} = \mu_{\overline{X}} = \mu(mu)\zeta_{\overline{X}} = \overline{X}$$

$$\overline{X} = \mu = \frac{\sum_{i=1}^{n} X_i}{n}$$

$$\text{Limits}_{\overline{X}} = \mu \pm (3 \div \sqrt{m})\sigma_X$$

$$= \mu \pm 3 \text{ standard deviations} = \mu \pm 3\sigma$$

The range (R) in the simplest terms is the largest measurement minus the smallest measurement. In the example stated originally, R = 1.41 − 1.08 = 0.33. The smaller the range, the less variability is involved. Consider the distribution range in the graphs in Figure 11-15.

The statistics of an R chart involve the use of some constants found in Figure 11-16, which is based on normal populations.

(*Text continues on p. 232.*)

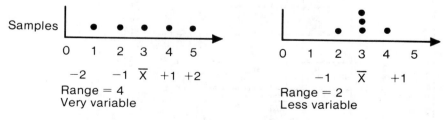

Fig. 11-15.   Range = distribution.

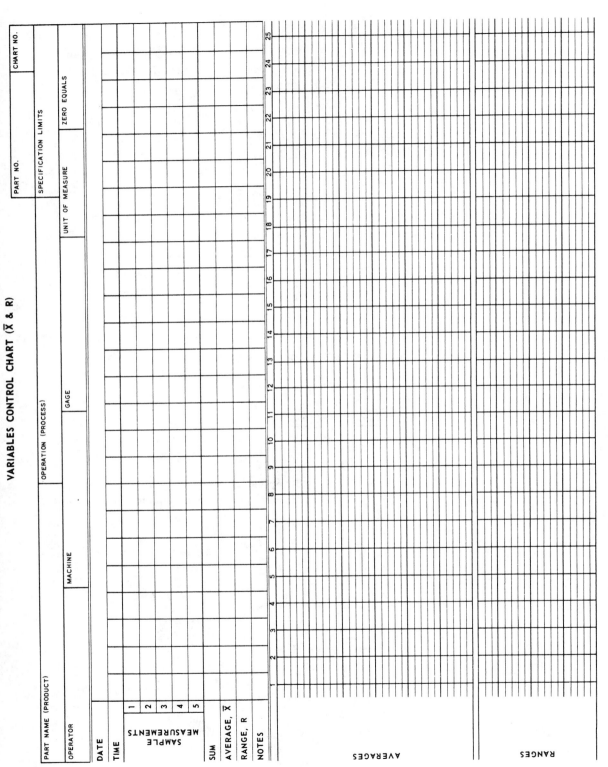

Fig. 11-16. Variables control chart.

230

CONTROL LIMITS

SUBGROUPS INCLUDED _____

$\bar{R} = \dfrac{\Sigma R}{k} =$

$\bar{\bar{X}} = \dfrac{\Sigma \bar{X}}{k} =$

or

$\bar{X}'$ (MIDSPEC. OR STD.) =

$A_2\bar{R} =$ x

$UCL_{\bar{x}} = \bar{\bar{X}} + A_2\bar{R}$ =

$LCL_{\bar{x}} = \bar{\bar{X}} - A_2\bar{R}$ =

$UCL_R = D_4\bar{R} =$ x

LIMITS FOR INDIVIDUALS

COMPARE WITH SPECIFICATION OR TOLERANCE LIMITS

$\bar{\bar{X}}$ =

$\dfrac{3\bar{R}}{d_2} =$ x

$UL_x = \bar{\bar{X}} + \dfrac{3}{d_2}\bar{R}$ =

$LL_x = \bar{\bar{X}} - \dfrac{3}{d_2}\bar{R}$ =

US =

LS =

US - LS =

$6\sigma = \dfrac{6}{d_2}\bar{R}$ =

FACTORS FOR CONTROL LIMITS

n	A_2	D_4	d_2	$\dfrac{3}{d_2}$	A_M
2	1.880	3.268	1.128	2.659	0.779
3	1.023	2.574	1.693	1.772	0.749
4	0.729	2.282	2.059	1.457	0.728
5	0.577	2.114	2.326	1.290	0.713
6	0.483	2.004	2.534	1.184	0.701

MODIFIED CONTROL LIMITS FOR AVERAGES

BASED ON SPECIFICATION LIMITS AND PROCESS CAPABILITY. APPLICABLE ONLY IF: US - LS > 6σ.

US =

LS =

$A_M\bar{R} =$ x

$URL_{\bar{x}} = US - A_M\bar{R}$ =

$LRL_{\bar{x}} = LS + A_M\bar{R}$ =

Fig. 11-17. Calculation work sheet.

$$\text{Center line } \overline{R} = \complement_R = d_z \sigma X$$

$$\overline{R} = \frac{\Sigma R}{k}$$

$$k = \text{number of tests or samples}$$

$$\text{Upper control limit}_{\overline{R}} = UCL_R = D_4\overline{R}$$

$$\text{Lower control limit}_{\overline{R}} = LCL_R = D_3\overline{R}$$

Generally, for samples of six or less the lower control limit will be zero. So the R scale moves from zero to the upper limit (Figs. 11-16, 11-17, 11-18).

ANALYZE PAST DATA		CONTROL FROM STANDARDS, μ, σx
$\overline{X}$	• Average or mean	$\overline{x}$
$\overline{X} = \Sigma_i^r = 1\overline{X}/k$	Center line ($\complement$)	μ
$\overline{X} \pm A_2\overline{R}$ or $A_3\overline{s}$	Limits	$\mu \pm A\sigma x$
R	• Range	R
$\overline{R} = \Sigma_i^k/k$	Center line ($\complement$)	$d_2\sigma x$
$D_3\overline{R}, D_4\overline{R}$	Limits	$D_1\sigma x, D_2\sigma x$
s	• Standard deviation	s
$\overline{s}$	Center line ($\complement$)	$C_4\sigma x$
$B_3\overline{s}, B_4\overline{s}$	Limits	$B_5\sigma x, B_6\sigma x$

Estimate of measurement error (e) such as from a densitometer = $\overline{R} - d_2$ or $\overline{s} - C_4$

$$\text{Variance } = \frac{\Sigma_{i=1}^{N} (Xi - \mu)^2}{N}$$

$$\text{Sample variance } = s^2 = \frac{(X_i - \overline{X})^2}{n - 1}$$

$$\text{Standard deviation, population} = \sigma = \sigma^2$$

$$\text{sample} = \sqrt{\sigma^2} = \sqrt{\frac{\Sigma (X_i - \overline{X})^2}{n - 1}}$$

Cumulative Sum Charts

A more sophisticated analysis is provided by working with cumulative sum (cusum) charts, which are, like a Shewhart chart, a type of sequential analysis based on data gathered. A quality characteristic such as speed (Q_s) is followed in relation to a standard quality value ($Q_o - s$).

$$\text{Cusum } (Q_s) = \Sigma_k = 1(Q_i - Q_o - s)$$

Sample Size n	Factors for Control limits for $\bar{x}$			Factors for Standard deviations, s		Factors for control limits for s				Factors for ranges R		Factors for control limits for R			
n	A	A_2	A_3	c_4	c_5	B_3	B_4	B_5	B_6	d_2	d_3	D_1	D_2	D_3	D_4
2	2.121	1.880	2.659	.798	.603	0	3.267	0	2.606	1.128	.853	0	3.686	0	3.267
3	1.732	1.023	1.954	.886	.463	0	2.568	0	2.276	1.693	.888	0	4.358	0	2.575
4	1.500	.729	1.628	.921	.389	0	2.266	0	2.088	2.059	.880	0	4.698	0	2.282
5	1.342	.577	1.427	.940	.341	0	2.089	0	1.964	2.326	.864	0	4.918	0	2.115
6	1.225	.483	1.287	.952	.308	.030	1.970	.029	1.874	2.534	.848	0	5.078	0	2.004
7	1.134	.419	1.182	.959	.282	.118	1.882	.113	1.806	2.704	.833	.205	5.203	.076	1.924
8	1.061	.373	1.099	.965	.262	.185	1.815	.179	1.751	2.847	.820	.387	5.307	.136	1.864
9	1.000	.337	1.032	.969	.246	.239	1.761	.232	1.707	2.970	.808	.546	5.394	.184	1.816
10	.949	.308	.975	.973	.232	.284	1.716	.276	1.669	3.078	.797	.687	5.469	.223	1.777
11	.905	.285	.927	.975	.221	.321	1.679	.313	1.637	3.173	.787	.812	5.534	.256	1.744
12	.866	.266	.886	.978	.211	.354	1.646	.346	1.610	3.258	.778	.924	5.592	.284	1.716
13	.832	.249	.850	.979	.202	.382	1.618	.374	1.585	3.336	.770	1.026	5.646	.308	1.692
14	.802	.235	.817	.981	.194	.406	1.594	.399	1.563	3.407	.762	1.121	5.693	.329	1.671
15	.775	.223	.789	.982	.187	.428	1.572	.421	1.544	3.472	.755	1.207	5.737	.348	1.652
16	.750	.212	.763	.983	.181	.448	1.552	.440	1.526	3.532	.749	1.285	5.779	.364	1.636
17	.728	.203	.739	.985	.175	.466	1.534	.458	1.511	3.588	.743	1.359	5.817	.379	1.621
18	.707	.194	.718	.985	.170	.482	1.518	.475	1.496	3.640	.738	1.426	5.854	.392	1.608
19	.688	.187	.698	.986	.165	.497	1.503	.490	1.483	3.689	.733	1.490	5.888	.404	1.596
20	.671	.180	.680	.987	.161	.510	1.490	.504	1.470	3.735	.729	1.548	5.922	.414	1.586
21	.655	.173	.663	.988	.157	.523	1.477	.516	1.459	3.778	.724	1.606	5.950	.425	1.575
22	.640	.167	.647	.988	.153	.534	1.466	.528	1.448	3.819	.720	1.659	5.979	.434	1.566
23	.626	.162	.633	.989	.150	.545	1.455	.539	1.438	3.858	.716	1.710	6.006	.443	1.557
24	.612	.157	.619	.989	.147	.555	1.445	.549	1.429	3.895	.712	1.759	6.031	.452	1.548
25	.600	.153	.606	.990	.144	.565	1.435	.559	1.420	3.931	.709	1.804	6.058	.459	1.541

Formulas for Control Charts for Variables, $\bar{x}$, s, R

Purpose of Chart	Chart for	Central Line	3-sigma Control Limits
No Standard Given - used for analyzing past data for control. ($\bar{x}$, $\bar{R}$, $\bar{s}$ are average values for data being analyzed.)	Averages, $\bar{x}$	$\bar{\bar{x}}$	$\bar{\bar{x}} \pm A_2\bar{R}$, or $\bar{\bar{x}} \pm A_3\bar{s}$ $D_3\bar{R}, D_4\bar{R}$ $B_3\bar{s}, B_4\bar{s}$
	Ranges, R	$\bar{R}$	
	Std. Devs., s	$\bar{s}$	
Standards Given - Used for controlling quality with respect to standards given μ, σ. $R'_n = d_2\sigma$ for n.	Averages, $\bar{x}$	μ	$\mu \pm A\sigma$
	Ranges, R	$d_2\sigma$ or R'_n	$D_1\sigma, D_2\sigma$ $D_3R'_n, D_4R'_n$
	Std. devs., s	$c_4\sigma$	$B_5\sigma, B_6\sigma$

$E(s) = c_4\sigma$, $\sigma_s = c_5\sigma$, $E(R) = d_2\sigma$, $\sigma_R = d_3\sigma$.

Fig. 11-18.   Control chart constants for averages $\bar{X}$, standard deviations (s), and ranges (R), from normal populations. Factors for computing central lines and three sigma control limits.

If $Q_o - s$ (the speed point standard) in an average value for speed, cusum (Q_s) will remain close to zero; but if the $Q_o - s$ is different, the sum (Q_s) will rapidly move away from center. The object here is to aim for a target and to have a system that quickly and accurately indicates when there is movement away from the aim. How sharply the data slope away is important in the analysis. A V-shaped mask is required for all calculations. The mask is not difficult to construct or to use. There is packaged software available for most personal computers. Keep in mind that Shewhart charts show general homogeneity: there is control with some variation; out of control is due to some assignable cause. Cusum presents a very quick indication of deviation from the standard.

In summary, statistical trend charts are charts of data dealing with the control of some quality standard and offer both more accurate interpretation and additional information than practical trend charts. Statistical trend charts require some additional testing to increase the sample size, sometimes called the cell size. A minimum of twice daily or twice per period such as a shift is suggested, with three times being significantly better because of the nature of the radiographic business. Because radiography is a business, the best methods should be employed to ensure the best product for the least cost. Statistical quality control, of which trend charts are the foundation, is in its essence an economic tool. It is strongly suggested that all radiography departments institute some sort of quality control. Those who have a solid program should elevate to Shewhart charts, at least for the speed measurement. Those with modified or complete Shewhart ($\overline{X}$, R) charts should consider cusum.

Plotting Trend Charts

Measurement Values

One of the difficulties of interpreting charts lies in the incorrect or incomplete establishment and maintenance of the charts. Always remember that charts are a history, a growth record, a running record, a graphic display. If the history is flawed or the picture sketchy, the observer has trouble visualizing the picture. Sensitometrically, only four values are measureable:

D_{max} or BKGD
Contrast
Speed
D_{min}

D_{max} means maximum density for the maximum exposure, but since the film may not have received a truly maximum exposure, the true maximum density has not been reached. Because of this confusion, the term *background density* (BKGD) is often used. If D_{max} relates to the maximum exposure given, then it is accurate.

Contrast is a difference between two densities and may be measured in a variety of positions on the H&D curve or may simply be the difference of densities of two steps on a gray scale. The measurement derived from drawing the H&D curve is considered a calculation. The measurement derived from reading two steps and subtracting the densities is an indicated value. Contrast levels are calculated as follows:

	Calculated Coordinates	Indicated
Medical	Toe: $(0.25 + B + F)$, $(1.00 + B + F)$	Speed point–D of 2 steps lower
	Mid: $(1.00 + B + F)$, $(2.00 + B + F)$	2 steps above speed–speed point
	Upper: $(2.00 + B + F)$, $(3.00 + B + F)$	
	Average gradient: $(0.25 + B + F)$ $(2.00 + B + F)$	2 steps above speed–2 steps below speed
	Gamma: Straight-line portion slope	2 steps above speed–speed point
	Gradient point: Tangent to any point	
Industrial	Gross: (1.00), (3.00)	1 step above speed–speed point
	Net (ANSI): $(1.50 + B + F)$, $(3.50 + B + F)$	

Speed is a measure of film sensitivity and is defined as the measure of energy needed to produce a specified density on the film. This specified density is

$$\text{Medical:} \quad 1.00 + B + F$$

$$\text{Industrial:} \quad 2.00 + B + F$$

Since the controlled film is given a controlled exposure, this is an excellent tool for gauging processing consistency. Indicated values may be obtained by eyeballing a fifth root of two gray scale (Du Pont ELS sensitometer) or by measuring the density on that step of the gray scale that is closest, but above the desired speed point.

D_{min} is the minimum density recorded for the minimum exposure. In medical radiography, this is often coincidentally equal to B + F values. However, B + F is inherent; D_{min} is the result of an exposure. If they are equal, it is truly a coincidence and the two should not be confused. In general photography and the specialty areas, which use more basic photographic techniques, there is a general rule that D_{min} must be about OD.30 above B + F to ensure adequate exposure. Usually, most institutions plot B + F in place of D_{min} and/or use the terms interchangeably. This is adequate initially but should eventually be converted to D_{min}. B + F is inherent in the film.

It is the result of manufacturing, shipping, and storage. Assuming that all of these factors are normal, then B + F becomes a rather stoic value uninfluenced by processing variables. Quality control personnel are often confronted by a virtual straight-line B + F chart along with wildly changing speed and contrast, but this is to be expected. All too often too much emphasis or weight is placed on B + F values.

Calculated versus Indicated

Calculated values must come from an H&D curve (Fig. 11-19). An exception would be some of the computer software available that allows the posting of density readings. The computer does all of the calculations with or without the drawing of the curve. Calculations are more accurate and may be required under various codes or specifications. For quality control charts, at least initially, indicated values are usually adequate. Part of the reason why indicated values are useful is that they easily allow for an adequate quality measurement (there is both subjective and objective error factors involved). Quality control is relatively new to radiography, and management generally has not allocated sufficient personnel hours to permit multiple tests or complete testing. As a result, indicated values, where permitted, allow data to be rapidly gathered. If several tests are made, the accuracy improves. Calculated values might be made on a random sampling basis or as a periodic cross-check. However, if possible, by all means make calculations. Indicated values are also called indexes.

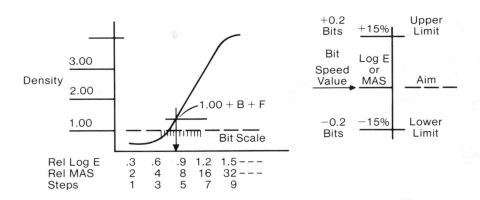

Calculated Speed: Exposure to produce a density of 1.00 less fog
Bit Speed Coordinate (1.00 + B +F), Bit Speed
Scale on Du Pont Graph Paper
(Step 11 = 16.0 Bits, Step 9 = 17.0 Bits,
etc.) Converts to Arithmetic Values.

Fig. 11-19.   Calculated speed and chart construction.

Setting up Charts

Speed could be an indicated value where the step on the master film gray scale closest to the speed point (medical = 1.00, industrial = 2.00) is read and plotted. The chart would have an aim or midpoint and a plus and a minus value. The plus and minus values would be a 15% density deviation (D ±0.15) for medical and 20% for industrial (D ±0.20). The technician (quality control personnel) reads the appropriate step on a densitometer and records the reading on the chart. The chart may be stated in a percent scale or density scale (Fig. 11-20).

The Du Pont Cronex sensitometer for medical and cine applications contains a portion of a fifth root of two exposure scale. The fifth root of two $(5\sqrt{2})$ is a number, 1.15, which indicates the exposure increments. Step to step represents a 15% exposure change. Because this is such a narrow range $(\sqrt{2} = 41\%$ step to step, $\times 2 = 100\%$ step to step) a test film may be visually, accurately compared to a master to determine a match or a percentage difference. The chart would be set up for indicated percent change or step difference (one step equals 15%) Figure 11-21 shows examples of visual comparisons.

Contrast charts, whether based on indicated or calculated value, will be set up with an aim and usually a range of ±10%. The chart should be properly and completely labeled.

B + F is very insensitive and is charted as density readings. D_{max} tends to be oversensitive in that it has greater variability but little influence on subject image quality. For this reason, it is seldom plotted. If it is plotted as a density reading, then ±20% would be the range.

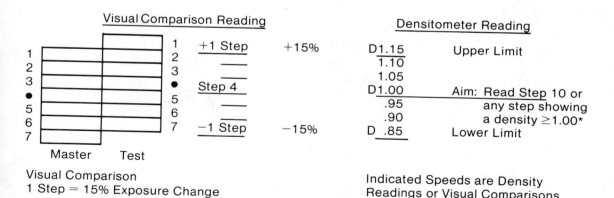

Visual Comparison Reading

1	+1 Step	+15%
2	—	
3	—	
•	Step 4	
5	—	
6	—	
7	−1 Step	−15%

Master Test

Visual Comparison
1 Step = 15% Exposure Change

Densitometer Reading

D1.15 — Upper Limit
1.10
1.05
D1.00 — Aim: Read Step 10 or
.95 any step showing
.90 a density ≥1.00*
D .85 — Lower Limit

Indicated Speeds are Density
Readings or Visual Comparisons

*Read: Density equal to or greater than one.

Fig. 11-20. Indicated speed and chart construction.

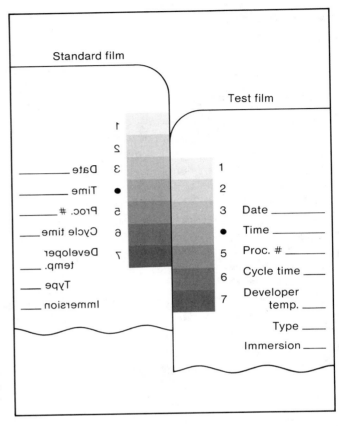

Fig. 11-21.   Visual comparison strip based on fifth root of two-exposure scale.

Points to Plot

Just as three tests per shift or work period supply a better data base, a better sample, a better picture than one a day, so does plotting multiple points (speed, contrast, D_{max}, B + F, D_{min}, and/or temperature) help to paint a better picture. Even when only speed is plotted, adding an R chart and other data will help in the interpretation. In the chart sequence shown in Figure 11-22, it is easy to see how increasing information aids interpretation. Chart A shows a single-point plot. We see stable but rising speed. The trend is toward the out-of-limits, out of control upper limit. What is the most likely cause? Was there another variable at play that is not known about, such as the time of day the test was made? The data block should be filled in. In chart B, the temperature chart is included to form a dual-point chart. Any second point could have been charted, but temperature is a good choice because it directly influences speed. From the chart, it might be concluded that temperature is stable and is not the cause of the speed increase. Thus,

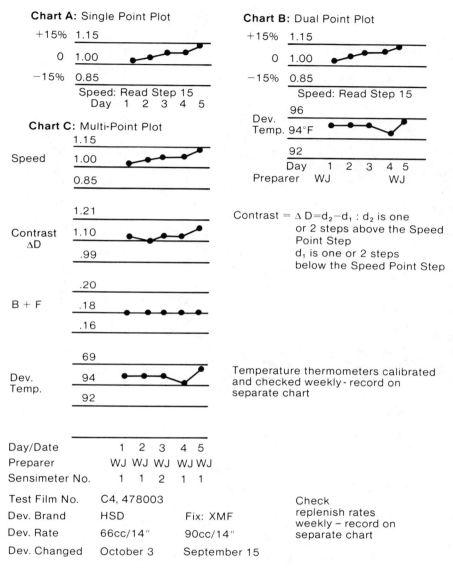

Chart A: Single Point Plot

Chart B: Dual Point Plot

Speed: Read Step 15

Contrast $= \Delta D = d_2 - d_1$: d_2 is one or 2 steps above the Speed Point Step

d_1 is one or 2 steps below the Speed Point Step

Temperature thermometers calibrated and checked weekly - record on separate chart

Check replenish rates weekly – record on separate chart

Day/Date	1	2	3	4	5
Preparer	WJ	WJ	WJ	WJ	WJ
Sensimeter No.	1	1	2	1	1

Test Film No.	C4, 478003		
Dev. Brand	HSD	Fix: XMF	
Dev. Rate	66cc/14″	90cc/14″	
Dev. Changed	October 3	September 15	

Fig. 11-22.   Single versus multipoint plots.

one must look elsewhere. Perhaps the time factor but more likely the replenishment rate (chemical activity) is incorrect. Again check the data block for the test person's initials, the time, date, etc. They are blank! Much information and confidence have been gained by adding just one extra test point. Interpretation is easier, is more complete, and may be more accurate. In chart C is found a multiple-point chart that is actually multiple charts. A true multipoint chart would have three or more test values plotted on the same chart, a very confusing situation that is to be avoided. Even with additional information, the cause of the speed rise may not be better understood. However, one valid conclusion is that since nothing seems to be causing it, it is probably normal fluctuation and most likely will return toward the center line. Further testing would confirm or reject this hypothesis. In studying sensitometry, it is learned that fog is noninformational density that has two obvious effects: It raises speed and lowers contrast. What can cause B + F to rise? It could be temperature and usually is, except that the chart states that the temperature is correct. Perhaps the chart is correct but the thermometer is lying, broken, or was misread. Another cause of fog could be adverse storage conditions: too long (age), pressure, heat, and/or moisture. Perhaps stray radiation preexposed the film. Maybe a different film emulsion was used in place of the set-aside test film. A good quality control technician is one who takes the bait and becomes curious about the signals and tries to solve the riddle. Remember the two major errors of any type of chart (practical or statistical): taking action when none is required and missing the opportunity to take action when required or to learn from a situation. Compare these charts to yours. A stranger should be able to review your charts and come to the same conclusions. What could or should be added to the data bank, the background information in chart C?

Remember that a basic radiographic quality control program includes these four steps:

1. Expose
2. Develop
3. Measure
4. Interpret

If the processor is being monitored, then the film is set aside and the exposure is as reproducible as possible. If the generator is being tested, the film is set aside and processing is controlled so that the effects of different exposures may be judged. Measurement should involve a densitometer that is zeroed and verified in calibration. It is insufficient simply to zero the equipment. Interpretation is the reason why all of the other work or steps are being made. How much information is needed to make decisions, to interpret what is happening? The answer will vary by department. However, do not overlook or cast aside information unless it is proved to be of no value. Consider film brand, film type, film emulsion number, sensitometer number, wash temperature, wash flow rate, chemical replenishment rate, cleaning schedule, testing personnel, processor operation, dryer temperature, ambient temperature and humidity, day of week, day of month, work load, standby hours, exposure device, film expiration date, film storage conditions (central and darkrooms), etc. These items could be identified and recorded. Many of them could be charted.

Number of Tests per Period (Shift or Day)

In an industrial facility such as a nuclear power station, there may be a large batch of films processed at the end of one shift when welders finish. There is no leeway for error, no chance to repeat the exposure before the second shift of welders starts up. This places a unique demand on quality control. There is extra pressure to ensure consistency during specified peak periods. Surprisingly, this occurs in medical facilities all the time and is so routine that it is not noticed. Most medical facilities process 75% of a processor's daily work load during the first 3 or 4 hours, from 8:00 AM to noon. Only in some industrial labs is a steady flow found, and that usually is around the clock. In those cases, each shift keeps its own charts. But for the ebb and flow of a typical radiography department, testing must be done before and after the high-production period. High volume and a very small error in replenishment rates, for example, will show a cumulative effect that can be dramatic in a short period. The following chart analyzes the work load and makes suggestions based on the conditions. Testing halfway through a production period is useless, is not a valid quality control technique, and may mask serious problems. Testing until a good result is finally obtained so the chart looks correct is an unacceptable approach.

	Tests Per Day Or Shift			
Time period	7 AM–12 PM	12 PM–4 PM	4 PM–12 AM	12 AM–7 AM
Films processed	300	100	10–50	0–20
Run test	7 AM	12 PM	4 PM	7 AM
Shift testing	7 AM, 3 PM		3 PM, 11 pm	11 PM, 7 AM

In every test, there is the specter of error in an unassigned variable. By doing multiple testing, error may be negated (Fig. 11-23).

Notice in the chart of two tests per day that there is low activity each morning followed by increased activity, except on day 15. This is not unusual, since it is showing the effects of overnight developer oxidation followed by a high replenishment rate as the result of the morning high-volume period. Note that the chart of one test per day looks like an average of the two-tests chart—but is it? Can false assumptions be made from the one-test chart? Most people respond in the affirmative and are positively receptive to the increased information gained from the second chart because a better picture emerges. Consider the three-test-per-day chart and notice immediately that starting on day 13 there are six test points trending upward. Normally, when five data points in sequence indicate a trend, there is indeed a trend and action should be taken. It is helpful, when reviewing the third chart, to know that the

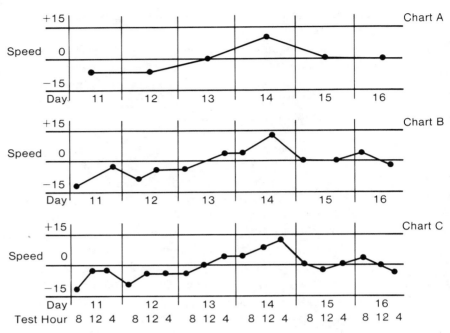

Fig. 11-23.   Multiple tests versus single tests.

processor operates 24 hours continuously on days 11 and 12 whereas on days 13, 14, and 15 it operates only 12 hours. The chart shows the effect of low-volume aerial oxidation on days 11 and 12. These 2 days are in control because of the chosen replenishment rate, which was selected based on the needs of the film and also to help fight aerial oxidation. Days 13, 14, and 15 have reduced film volume and reduced aerial oxidation but the same re-plenishment rate, so activity migrates upward. Perhaps the day 15 fall-back, although perfectly acceptable, is due to low film volume so that aerial oxi-dation again becomes a problem. Maybe tests should be done on day 16 (Saturday), when there is extremely low volume. Maybe tests on Sunday will show why Monday is always at a low activity level.

Treatment of Multiple Test Data

In the chart shown in Figure 11-24, tests are made each day at 8 AM, noon, and 4 PM and are plotted. Each day is treated differently. Day 1 joins together the plots and creates a track of how the process is shifting; it makes no assumptions or adjustments. Day 2 has created an arbitrary average, which may be misleading in that the track may look better or worse than it really is. Day 3 to day 4 has chosen to track the midpoints, which is another form of averaging. Notice that it suggests no variability, while the ignored data points indicate there is loss of activity every morning. Days 5 and 6 are the

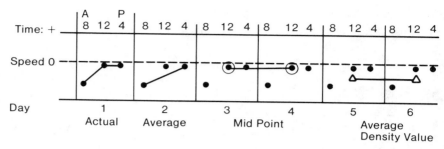

Fig. 11-24.   Multiple test data.

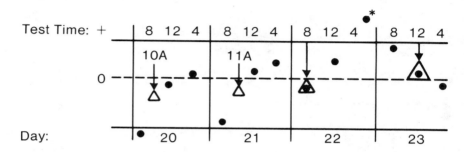

▲ = Arbitrary tests, one/day
● = Specific tests, on time three/day

*Out of limits, correction made by lowering temperature 2°F, new test made and recorded.

Fig. 11-25.   Testing on time.

plot of the mathematical average and make the chart very confusing. If She-whart charts are used, then the three daily tests would be a sample and the average value would be plotted on the $\overline{X}$ chart. The range (R) of variability would be calculated. However, if the practical chart method is used and the raw data are plotted, then no assumptions or averaging should be made. The track should follow the data as in day 1. It shows best the day-to-day and within-day variations. The same would be true of weekly trends also.

Testing on Time

In the chart shown in Figure 11-25, another consideration is made regarding testing and work schedules. Frequently the quality control technician begins to test several pieces of equipment on time but is distracted so that a scheduled test becomes an unscheduled test. A word of caution: If the distraction is an emergency process failure (exposure, film, holders, processors), this is a clear indication of quality out of control and a failure in the overall quality assurance program. There is a very low degree of assurance when the system fails. The more failures, the less effective is the program. Remember, quality control personnel and programs exist to prevent, not to fix. In analyzing the chart, we see the same process monitored three times a day at exact times ($\pm$15 minutes). The arbitrary test times on an unscheduled basis are contrived but make a very important point. The arbitrary tests are 10 AM on day 20, 11 AM on day 21, 8 AM on day 22, and noon on day 23. The one test per day at different times suggests excellent consistency over the 4 days. The three tests per day at the scheduled times indicate that a serious, out-of-control problem might occur (based on day 20, 21 increase and pattern) and did occur at 4 PM on day 22. Action must be taken so that the process can function reasonably well on day 23 at 8 AM. A correction was made. The once-a-day arbitrary test showed no problems or changes. Charts are kept to provide inferences, not to hide them, and to provide a chance to make the correct decision, not to obviate the need for decisions.

Recording Data

Record what is measured or seen. If densitometric readings are made, the procedure is to zero and verify calibration of the densitometer. Read B + F and the various steps on the gray scale. Always try to remain in the physical center of the step for greatest accuracy. Whether the scale is the result of ionizing radiation or a step tablet and light, there tend to be bell-shaped distribution curves in a biaxial mode (Fig. 11-26).

To construct an H & D curve, start at the low densities and read to the higher densities if reading all steps. When a densitometric reading is made, record the reading and do not make a second one unless the first is very peculiar. The reason for making a single test is that there is error in the densitometer expressed as accuracy ($\pm$0.02) and reproducibility ($\pm$0.02). The same film density might read differently the second the time because of inaccuracy and/or nonreproducibility. The third reading might be the same as the first but may also be due to the same conditions but reverse combinations that affect the second reading. Perhaps as a separate experiment, quality control personnel should read across a single step in two directions to locate the center, draw a small circle, and read that density 10 times. The next day read the small circle 10 times again. The real variability of a densitometer is small and of little influence on our judgment of quality or of control, but it cannot be ignored. Thus, the reading that is obtained is recorded, knowing that if a slight fluctuation is seen it may indeed be due to the densitometer. The chart must be set up so that small density increments can easily be recorded. A chart set up with lines labeled D 1.00, 1.10, 1.20, etc. would not allow for proper display. It would also compress the data so that variability would appear as demonstrated in Figure 11-27.

When making a visual comparison using the fifth root of a two-exposure

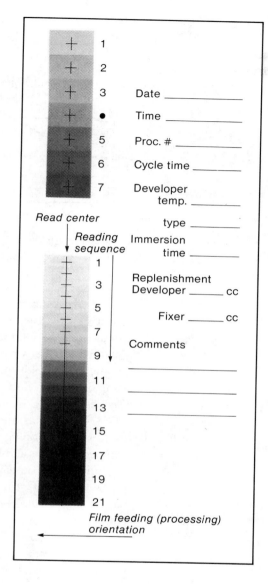

Fig. 11-26. Proper orientation of gray scale for processing and densitometer reading.

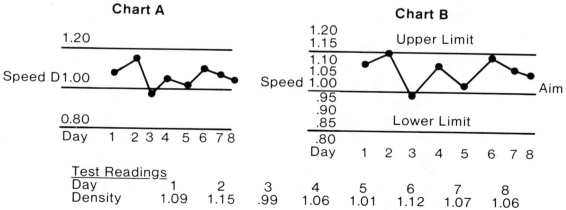

Fig. 11-27. Setting the proper scale spacing to avoid distortion.

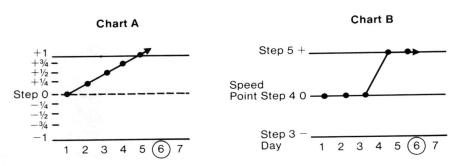

Fig. 11-28.   Visual interpretation recording.

scale between a test and a master film (never test film to test film) read and record your estimate. If it is estimated that there is a half or slightly less than half a step difference, it should be recorded as a quarter step change and not as a half step. If there is half step darker test film, do not try to force the data into a pattern by analyzing whether a half step is bad or good. Some people would plot the half step as no change, and others would plot the same data as a full step. What should be displayed is what the best estimate, the best reading is: Always record what is measured, as shown in Figure 11-28. Chart A has the data recorded the way it was read. It is obvious that there is a developing trend. The inference is that additional testing and/or compensation should be made because every indication points to an out-of-control process on day 6. Chart B represents the same data forced into neat pockets of "okay" (midpoint) or out one step (upper limit). Based on the data in chart B, the conclusion is that although days 4 and 5 are at the upper control limit, the process has not exceeded the limit, appears to be stable, and day 6 will be the same as day 5. This last conclusion is based on the "fact" that days 1, 2, and 3 were flat. It is logical to expect the next 3-day period to be equally flat, at a higher level. This is a correct assumption based on false data. Remember the two problem aspects of charts: taking action when none is required and failing to take action when required.

Tracking

When the various test results are placed on the initial chart as dots, there develops a variety of errors and much confusion about how to handle this display. The dots should be large enough to be seen easily. They should be accurately positioned. The spacing horizontally should be adequate for placing of dots. The space for a day should be wide enough to accommodate the tests performed. A chart should cover at least 1 week of time, and preferably a chart will cover 1 month. Always start a chart on the first of the month rather than running on day after day. The reason for these procedures is to aid in seeing trends within days, within weeks, and within months. People and business follow many cyclical patterns that they are often not aware of, and these could be an assignable cause of variability if identified.

Initially, a chart is set up with an arbitrary midpoint and an estimated acceptability range with upper and lower levels or limits (plus and minus). Shewhart believed the charts would show the technician how to set up the data. Indeed, prior to setting up a Shewhart chart, many tests should be made as previously discussed. However, all charts have to start someplace (aim) with a set of parameters (upper control limit, lower control limit). After a week or two or even a month, it may become apparent that the wrong aim or range was chosen. It may become obvious that the scale can be tightened down, as shown in Figure 11-29.

This consideration and adjustment may appear when the emulsion number for boxes of test film is changed. Remember that the goal is consistency and not finite values. Also, change must be understood and explainable.

This is not manipulation of the data, rather it is simply a response to the data that are giving indications of various values and variables. Certainly, if a nominal acceptable range is chosen and the data fly in and out of the range, then the system is out of control. The discussion here concerns the generally natural refinement in the charts as the process is better understood and the control improves, which is expected (Fig. 11-30).

Connecting dots can be an easy way to see trends, but if the tracking line from dot to dot is drawn freehand (permissible if there are multiple dots close together), there may be a false image of sloppiness in the process because that is what is seen. Dots should be connected from center to center with a straight edge. As can be seen in Figure 11-31, there are different chart qualities based on how the data are displayed, although all the data are iden-

Establishing Chart Aim and Modification with Experience

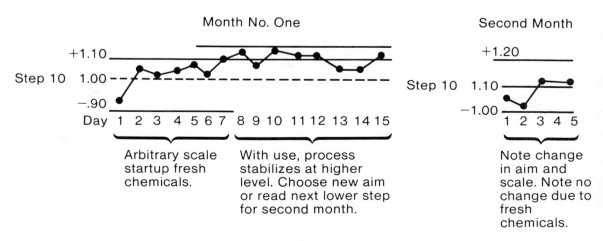

Fig. 11-29. Establishing chart aim and modification with experience.

tical. The fourth method (chart D) is somewhat tedious but effective. If the area below the dots is colored, a very dramatic graph would appear (chart E). Unfortunately, this would give the impression that they lay or varied between minus (LCL) and approximately the midpoint, and that is not the case since the data should flow around the midpoint. This type of chart looks falsely like an R chart, as does chart F. Example chart C is more correct and proper.

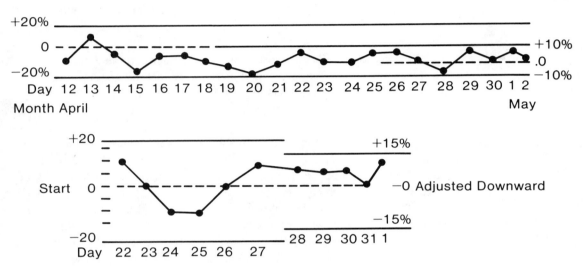

Fig. 11-30.   Establishing chart parameters (range) with experience.

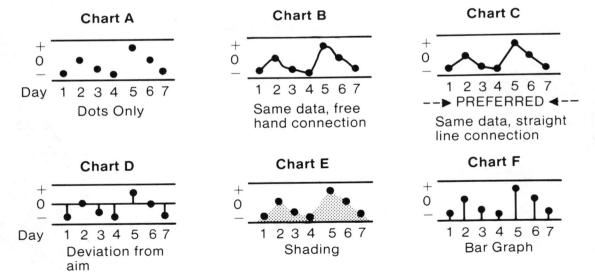

Fig. 11-31.   Charting styles.

Data points may only be connected together if they follow continuously. A very common mistake is either to leave out weekend spaces in a monthly chart or to join Friday to Monday, indicating some knowledge of the quality on Saturday and Sunday. First of all, tests should be made every day and recorded that day. Second, make no assumptions. If a gap appears in the data, it is left as a gap (Fig. 11-32).

Consider daily patterns in charting (Fig. 11-33). It would be easy to see a general rise in activity over the 3-day period (nine shifts), but notice that shift one is consistent each day (day 17 shows some up-and-down fluctuation that is normal). Shift two always starts low and shoots up. Shift three always falls. Based on the last test in shift three on day 19 and the first test on shift one of day 20, what is in store for the rest of day 20? Was the changing film volume noticed, and will that affect day 20? Sometimes it helps one's ability

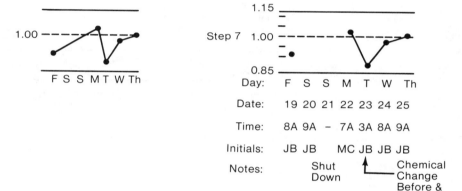

Fig. 11-32.   Complete versus incomplete data.

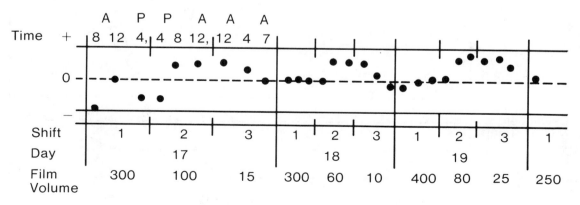

Fig. 11-33.   Daily shift patterns.

to see the trends if a different display is used or if the dots are connected together in groups or as a running record.

Compare the two charts in Figure 11-34 and see which shows the trends best. Both have the same data. There are weekly trends, week-to-week trends, and a monthly trend.

Figure 11-35 is an actual speed and developer temperature chart. It can be deduced that the speed increase on day 17 was not due to a temperature increase, because although the temperature chart shows a slight increase it is insignificant. Additional evidence is supplied as history. Note day 7, when

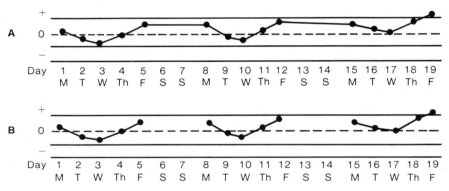

Fig. 11-34.   Seeing trends by proper plotting techniques.

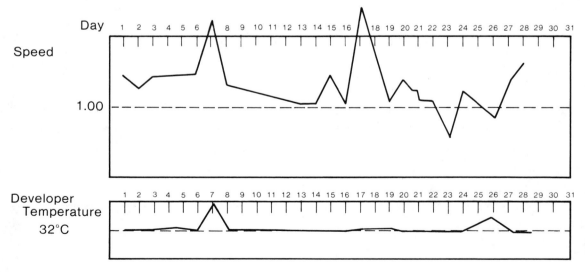

Fig. 11-35.   Handling out-of-limits: the essence of quality control.

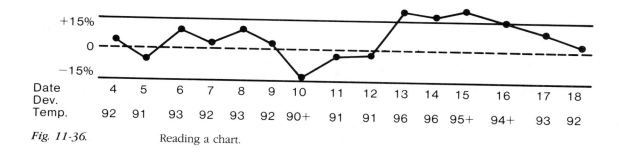

Date Dev.	4	5	6	7	8	9	10	11	12	13	14	15	16	17	18
Temp.	92	91	93	92	93	92	90+	91	91	96	96	95+	94+	93	92

Fig. 11-36.   Reading a chart.

the temperature went up and the speed responded by going noticeably higher. Thus, based on fact (temperature is okay) and history (day 7 cause and effect), temperature is not the cause—something else is. This is a false conclusion, however, because temperature was not measured or recorded on the dates in question. The plot line is jumping the gap, creating false, misleading data. Temperature may or may not be the cause. The chart, as drawn, creates confusion.

Figure 11-36 shows good control* from day 4 to day 13, with no alarms or signals. Day 13, however, is out of limits, beyond the range of acceptable quality. Because of previous data, this is not a process adjustment. This is, according to statistical quality control, an assignable variable gone wild, out of control, forcing the whole process out of control. There are two very important and simple concepts: out of control (or limits) and unacceptable. Whenever, and every time, a test point is outside the limits of acceptability, the system is out of control, quality is out of control, and something must be done. The first task is to retest. Next, test the electromechanical and chemical variables, which are the usually easy to measure controls of time, temperature, and replenishment. If a direct cause (temperature is up 2°, which is 15% exposure equivalent and film is 15% too dark) is found, correct it. If no cause is found, make a minor compensation to bring the process back, just inside the limits. While this work is being done, subsequent tests are being made and the results interpreted. This should all be recorded elsewhere. After control is regained, a test film confirms this and its data is recorded. The chart should show the problem test and the corrected test along with complete details. Trend charts are used precisely to tell when a system is out of control and to help make the right decisions. If the out-of-limits test is ignored, there is no control and there is no control program. Consider again the charts in Figures 11-36 and 11-37.

* Good control is achieved when there is a random fluctuation close to the midpoint or center line. There should not be a straight line or a sawtooth line. There should not be obvious repeating patterns or a continuous pattern. Any out-of-control system indicates bad control.

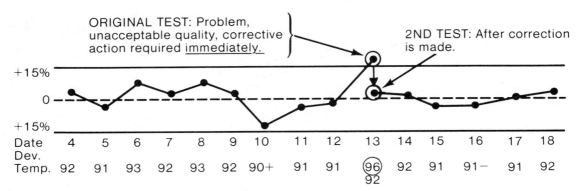

NOTES: Day 13, thermostat stuck. Contacts cleaned. Spare ordered on 7/14/86 JB.

Fig. 11-37.   Responding to chart signals and course correction.

Trend Chart Interpretation

Determining Optimal

A particular brand of chemistry may perform differently in two different processors. In any processor or processing system (including chemistry), the total effect of the electromechanics and chemistry on a piece of film with a controlled exposure is termed sensitometry and involves four measurements (D_{max}, contrast, speed, and D_{min}). How is optimal processing defined? How can trend charts be correctly interpreted? The answer lies in what a photographer refers to as a contrast response curve. For a range of developer immersion times, developer temperatures, and activities of developer, the various sensitometric values are measured. A narrow range will be found where contrast is maximum or optimal, and the best speed and D_{max} are achieved while keeping the fog level (D_{min}) unchanged. Since most radiographic processors have a fixed speed and chemicals are prepackaged, the major variable is temperature. In Figure 11-38, either indicated or calculated values could be used. This is a stylized drawing of actual data. It is clear that 92 to 94°F offers maximum contrast. At 93°F, the D_{max} (actually background density), maximum speed, and minimum fog are achieved for the maximum contrast. If temperature rises or falls, the contrast will decrease. However, since many people tend to underdevelop, we can look to the dashed line on the left and refer to this as normal. From this normal level, it can be predicted that as the temperature goes up or down not only will contrast go up and down but so will speed and D_{max}. Just the opposite occurs at the overdevelopment level of 96°F. Thus, based on a contrast response curve it is easy to predict what is happening when trend charts for speed and contrast are compared (Fig. 11-39). If they track together, there is general underdevelopment; if they track

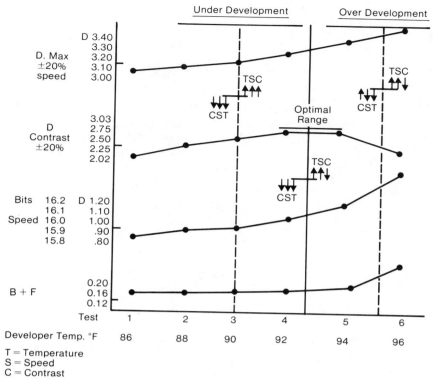

Fig. 11-38.   Contrast response chart: temperature response series.

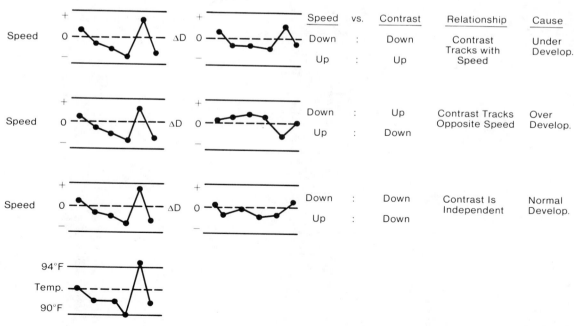

Fig. 11-39.   Trend chart interpretation based on response.

253

opposed, there is overdevelopment; if they track independently, there is good development. Remember that a certain chemical brand might perform differently in different processor brands. Each institution should perform its own contrast response curve series. Film manufacturer guidelines for processing are based on their analysis using this method. Also, personal preferences of the photo interpreter influence the final processing specifications. The Du Pont bit system for technique conversion of medical products has defined optimal processing as 15 bits with a ±15% (±0.2 bits) range of 14.8 to 15.2 bits. However, although all of this is important to understanding and is useful in establishing quality, it is also important in interpreting what is happening to the process.

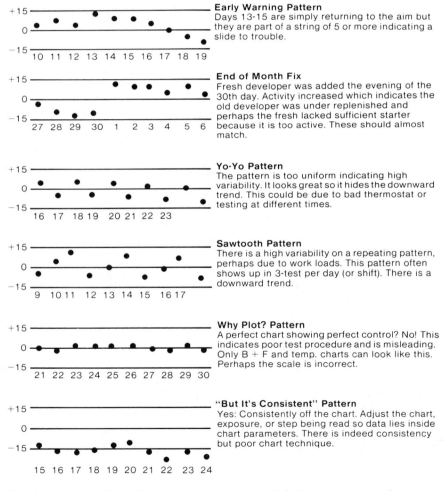

Early Warning Pattern
Days 13-15 are simply returning to the aim but they are part of a string of 5 or more indicating a slide to trouble.

End of Month Fix
Fresh developer was added the evening of the 30th day. Activity increased which indicates the old developer was under replenished and perhaps the fresh lacked sufficient starter because it is too active. These should almost match.

Yo-Yo Pattern
The pattern is too uniform indicating high variability. It looks great so it hides the downward trend. This could be due to bad thermostat or testing at different times.

Sawtooth Pattern
There is a high variability on a repeating pattern, perhaps due to work loads. This pattern often shows up in 3-test per day (or shift). There is a downward trend.

Why Plot? Pattern
A perfect chart showing perfect control? No! This indicates poor test procedure and is misleading. Only B + F and temp. charts can look like this. Perhaps the scale is incorrect.

"But It's Consistent" Pattern
Yes: Consistently off the chart. Adjust the chart, exposure, or step being read so data lies inside chart parameters. There is indeed consistency but poor chart technique.

Fig. 11-40.   Trend chart examples. (Connecting the dots may help in interpretation.)

Trend Chart Examples

In Figures 11-40 and 11-41, the dots should be connected using a ruler. This will make visualization easier and provide practice.

Trends in the Trend Chart

In Figure 11-42, there is nothing wrong with any portion of chart A. There is acceptable quality under control for all 30 days. However, control is tightened toward the end of the month.

Although Figure 11-42B shows very shallow data making the measurement technique suspect, it is possible to see weekly trends. Note the gradual increase in activity over the first 3 weeks. Note the trend back downward in the fourth week. Note weekly that day 1 is always very low activity. This is

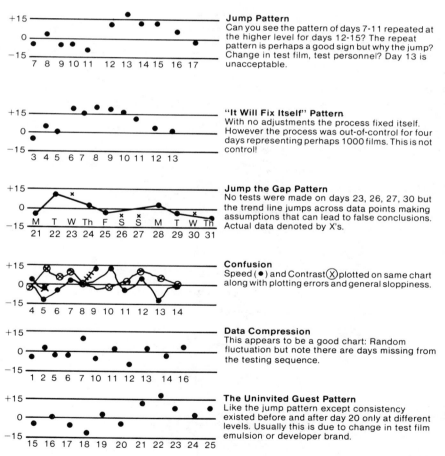

Jump Pattern
Can you see the pattern of days 7-11 repeated at the higher level for days 12-15? The repeat pattern is perhaps a good sign but why the jump? Change in test film, test personnel? Day 13 is unacceptable.

"It Will Fix Itself" Pattern
With no adjustments the process fixed itself. However the process was out-of-control for four days representing perhaps 1000 films. This is not control!

Jump the Gap Pattern
No tests were made on days 23, 26, 27, 30 but the trend line jumps across data points making assumptions that can lead to false conclusions. Actual data denoted by X's.

Confusion
Speed (●) and Contrast (X) plotted on same chart along with plotting errors and general sloppiness.

Data Compression
This appears to be a good chart: Random fluctuation but note there are days missing from the testing sequence.

The Uninvited Guest Pattern
Like the jump pattern except consistency existed before and after day 20 only at different levels. Usually this is due to change in test film emulsion or developer brand.

Fig. 11-41.   Trends in the trend chart.

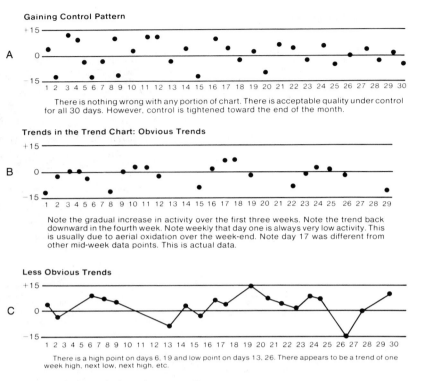

Gaining Control Pattern

A

There is nothing wrong with any portion of chart. There is acceptable quality under control for all 30 days. However, control is tightened toward the end of the month.

Trends in the Trend Chart: Obvious Trends

B

Note the gradual increase in activity over the first three weeks. Note the trend back downward in the fourth week. Note weekly that day one is always very low activity. This is usually due to aerial oxidation over the week-end. Note day 17 was different from other mid-week data points. This is actual data.

Less Obvious Trends

C

There is a high point on days 6, 19 and low point on days 13, 26. There appears to be a trend of one week high, next low, next high, etc.

Fig. 11-42.   Trends in the trend chart (continued).

usually a result of aerial oxidation over the weekend. Note that day 17 was different from other midweek data points. These are actual data.

Less Obvious Trends

There is a high point on days 6 and 19 and a low point on days 13 and 16 (Fig. 11-42C). There appears to be a trend of 1 week high, next low, next high, etc.

Speed and Contrast Tracking Together

The speed chart is the one used in Figure 11-42C. Here in Figure 11-43, it appears as drawn by the institution. There are procedural problems. Note that contrast tracks independently until day 20, when something happened such as contamination or temperature loss or tank level too low. The end of the month suggests underdevelopment, although contrast and speed are adequate.

Independent Tracking

Speed appears to make a distinct M pattern between days 7 and 9 and again between days 19 and 21 (Fig. 11-44). The data are somewhat confusing because of a failure to test each day and the jumping of gaps with the trend

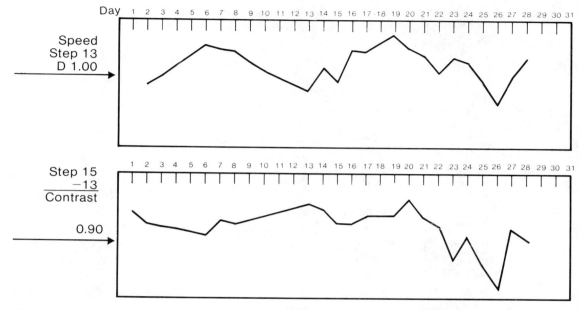

Fig. 11-43.   Speed and contrast tracking together.

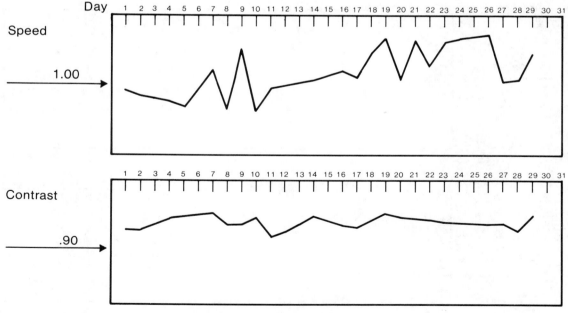

Fig. 11-44.   Independent tracking.

line. Note that speed is trending toward overdevelopment fog. Next month is going to be a problem unless controls are adjusted. Perhaps replenishment can be lowered 10%.

Contrast is independent of speed, indicating optimum development. There is a minor trend: Days 7 and 19 show high contrast points. This is mostly a coincidence. Note that there are two other high points that do not relate to speed changes.

Out of Control and Tracking Together

In Figure 11-45, speed is out of control 25% of the time (7 out of 28 test days). The upper limit on the chart is D 1.25, with the higher points hitting D 1.48 and 1.42, or 42% more density than should be on the film. Obviously something is wrong—or is it? Note that contrast tracks exactly like speed, indicating underdevelopment. But how can speed and contrast be too high if there is underdevelopment? Contamination by systems cleaners, weak developer hardener, or weak developer with temperature compensation are possible causes. Would it help to know that B + F is very high?

If speed is supposed to approximate D 1.00, there is lack of control. If speed is yet to be defined, then perhaps the range is approximately D 1.00 to D 1.30, where most of the data lie. The aim would be D 1.15. This is only slightly out of limits (but still unacceptable). Would last month's trend chart

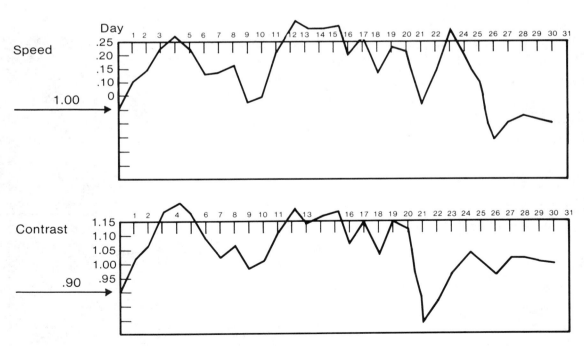

Fig. 11-45.   Out of control and tracking together.

help in determining if this processor is in control but high or if it is out of control?

Half-and-Half Pattern

In Figure 11-46, for the first 13 days speed and contrast are controlled. They appear independent of each other. However, perhaps you noticed the speed increase in the second week and the slight contrast increase.

Day 13 is out of control. Apparently it corrected itself, because no notes on tests or compensation were recorded. After day 13, note how suddenly speed and contrast begin tracking with each other. It is almost as if high temperature (speed rise) damaged the developer so that speed and contrast are marginal thereafter.

Note the wild swings in the last week of the month compared with the first week. The middle weeks are acceptably stable (except day 13). Would it be useful and important to you in making decisions to know that this processor produces the same wild swing in the last week of every month?

Half-Good/Half-Bad Pattern

In Figure 11-47, contrast has an aim of 0.90 but there is no indication of how this is derived. There are no scale markings. Contrast is very consistent, but its average (mean) is not 0.90 but closer to 1.5 units (seven lines) higher.

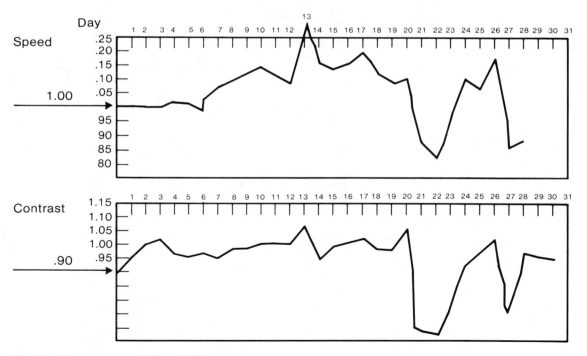

Fig. 11-46.   Half-and-half pattern.

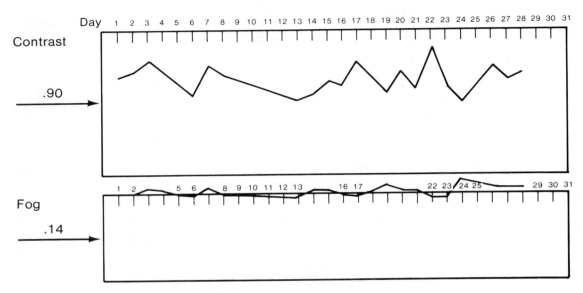

Fig. 11-47.   Half-good/half-bad pattern.

If each line is 0.01, then the average is along the 0.97 line. If each line is 0.02, then the average is 1.05. Thus, although contrast is well in control and there is a gentle roll of fluctuations, it is consistently about 10% higher than the aim.

The fog (B + F) is obviously at or off scale in an unacceptable range. The aim is D 0.14, but how that was chosen is not explained. Obviously the fog level is somewhere around D 0.18 (a few readings of 0.18 and 0.20 were written in). Setting the aim at 0.18 would place all of the data in the center of the chart, where they belong. To summarize, the fog is consistent and at an acceptable level but the charting indicates error and inconsistency.

Matched Processors?

In Figure 11-48A, the mean ($\overline{X}$) is 1.16, the median is 1.16, and the data are normally distributed (bell-shaped curve because mean and median are equal). The range is 1.00 to 1.27. Day 1 bit speed is 14.32, and day 31 bit speed is 14.43.

In Figure 11-48B, the mean ($\overline{X}$) is 1.20 and the median is 1.18. Distribution is skewed right (because of large high-value variables such as day 25). The range is 1.08 to 1.35. Day 1 bit speed is 14.49, and day 31 bit speed is 14.58. The following conclusions can be drawn:

- Both processors are approximately matched, with QC-1 R/T running about 7% more activity.
- Both processors are in control and consistent.
- Replotting M6-AN data on a chart with an aim of 1.20 will show a good

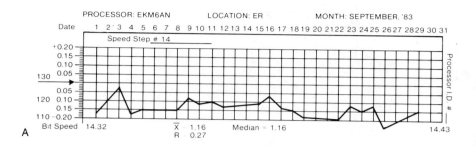

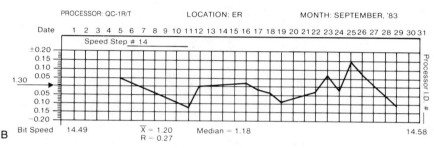

Fig. 11-48. Matched processors?

match to the QC-1 R/T. No other changes would be made, since units are indeed matched.

Almost Perfect

In Figure 11-49, a reproduction of actual data, both the test film emulsion and the chemistry were changed during the month. There appeared to be fairly complete support information, but there are some procedural problems. The numbers below are on the chart.

(1) There is confusion about the correct aim for speed. Apparently, the parenthetical number refers to the old emulsion number. (2) Apparently the new film was introduced on day 4. (3) The film on day 5 matches day 4 except that the speed point changed from 1.34 to 1.16, or a loss of 18% in density. The chart is misleading. At least this change in film occurred prior to the chemistry change on day 6. (4) The old chemistry and the new chemistry (5) have the same type of activity, and this is proved by the sensitometric values. (6) Note the rise in speed in the middle of the week. (7) There is good temperature stability the first week, but it rises 1°F the second week and is not recorded the third week when the speed increases (8). (9) Note that testing should be performed at 8:30 AM but ranged (10) from 7:45 AM to 10:00 AM. Certainly many films are processed before 10:00 AM. (11) Contrast is track-

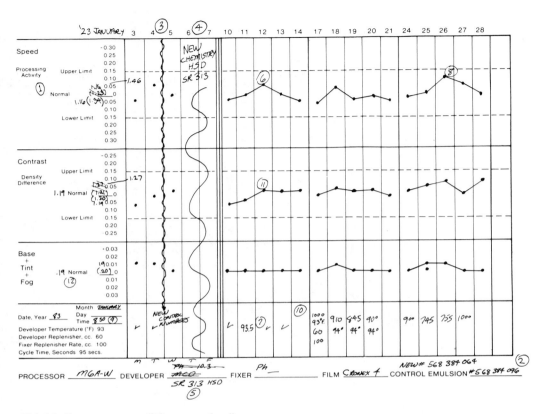

Fig. 11-49.   "Almost perfect."

ing with gentle swings, but note that it tracks with the speed in that there is a higher midweek period. (12) B + F is stable but seems to have influenced (or resulted from the same influence) as speed and contrast on day 18, since all three charts rise upward.

How can this chart be made less confusing? Would an examiner consider this chart to be professional documentation of a quality control function? Would the chart have to be explained to the examiner? Why the aim is changed so many times is unknown. There are a lot of data included, and despite two major changes (film and developer), there is good control. Perhaps the chart should look like one of those in Figure 11-50.

In Figure 11-51, all processors (four different ones, same month, same developer) would appear matched, since charts A, B, C, and D all show more or less a tendency for data to be in the center of the chart (disregard the wide fluctuations). But notice the aim points:

Chart A	1.21
B	1.12
C	1.17
D	1.13

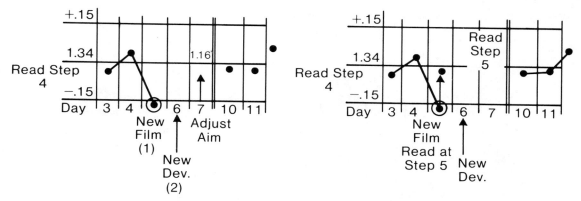

NOTES

(1) CRONEX 4 # 568384-096
    changed to
    CRONEX 4 # 568384-064 (new)
(2) CRONEX MCD changed to
    CRONEX HSD. 7 oz. starter used.

Fig. 11-50.   Correct chart adjustment to note film and chemical changes.

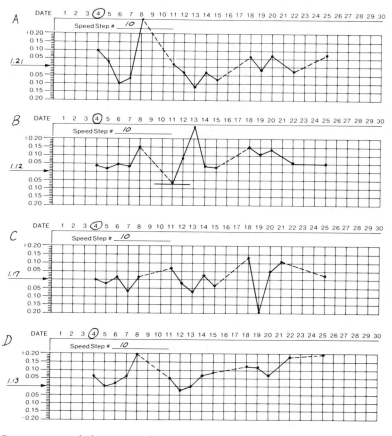

Fig. 11-51.   Processor trend chart examples.

Since the same step is read, this suggests that Chart C is in the middle, with chart A overdeveloping about 4% and chart B underdeveloping about 4%. The smallest to largest is only D 0.09, or about 9%. In other words, these charts all should have the same aim since they are so close.

Next let's consider the mean ($\overline{X}$) or average for the four charts and the ranges (R):

Chart	$\overline{X}$	R	Spread	±
A	1.21	1.09–1.28	19	10
B	1.12	1.05–1.27	22	11
C	1.17	0.97–1.30	33	16
D	1.13	1.13–1.32	19	10

Despite the wide fluctuations, the average of these four processors is virtually identical. The ranges are similar to chart C, having the biggest spread, and yet it looks relatively under control (which it is). All charts show a slight increase in speed toward the end of the month, but it is quite acceptable. Chart D looks like pending disaster. However, remember that the aim is 1.13, while the actual average is 1.20 and day 25 is reading 1.32, or about 12% higher than the average, which is less than the allowed 15% margin. If chart D is replotted using an aim of 1.20, it would appear acceptable.

In conclusion, these four processors are matched. Their charts should have the same aim point of 1.20. The wild fluctuations should have been controlled on days 8, 13, and 19 and actually were, according the institution's charts. These wild fluctuations become normal or reasonable if the aim point is adjusted as suggested above. For example, chart B, day 13 suggests disaster will occur, with all films coming out black. The data are off the chart. However, the density (speed point) is 1.27. If the chart aim were 1.20, this would amount to a meager 7% increase in density and would be of no consequence.

Complete Analysis Examples

Below are two complete analyses based on actual data from different hospitals. The charts are correctly constructed and complete. When interpreting charts, the object is to see if there is something worth investigating. Ideally, in a well-controlled process there might be no significant changes for months. Charts are useless unless they are reviewed to see if there are trends. Review the way the charts are set up and the analysis.

In Figure 11-52, everything is in control throughout the month, but there is a definite upward trend in speed B + F while contrast starts to fall. Since exposure and film are controlled, the cause must be processing, which has

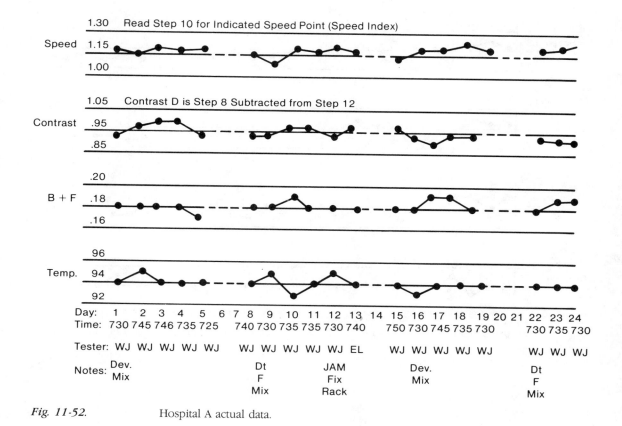

Fig. 11-52.   Hospital A actual data.

the variables time, temperature, and activity. Time should be checked to see if it is slowing down and increasing time in the developer, except that this would usually lead to equal or increased contrast. Temperature is not at fault, because the chart is stable. The developer may be too strong as a result of improper mixing (underdilution, improper sequence, or overmixing) or overreplenishment, or it may be slightly contaminated. If this pattern happens every month, then there is slight overreplenishment. Under some circumstances, contrast might have increased instead of decreasing for the same reason.

In Figure 11-53, there is loss of activity. Speed, contrast, and B + F all drop. It would appear that the new film is the cause, except that at the changeover there is only a small difference and this would not cause activity to fall off. Temperature is not at fault, nor is transport (it seldom speeds up). Finally, developer activity loss must be suspected. This is probably due to underreplenishment. If the level in the developer tank is low, there would be less development time. However, it is hard to imagine why the tank would be gradually losing chemicals.

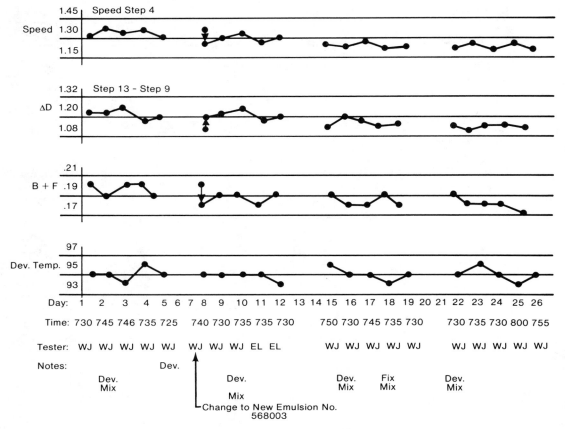

Fig. 11-53.   Hospital B actual data.

Other Factors That Could Be Charted

Figure 11-54 shows a variety of different items or subjects that could be charted. Note that the aim and scale change depending on the subject being monitored. Each chart is set up as any chart should be. The dots are not connected, but that is left to the reader. A stick diagram could be used instead. Questions or observations are presented to help readers develop the practice of questioning.

Statistical Analysis

In the study charted in Figures 11-55 through 11-59, five processors were monitored for 1 month in a hospital. These are actual data. The processors were located in busy main diagnostic areas and low-volume special modality areas. The processors are labeled C1, C11, C21, C31, and C41, which happen to be the various columns used in a computer-based statistics package.

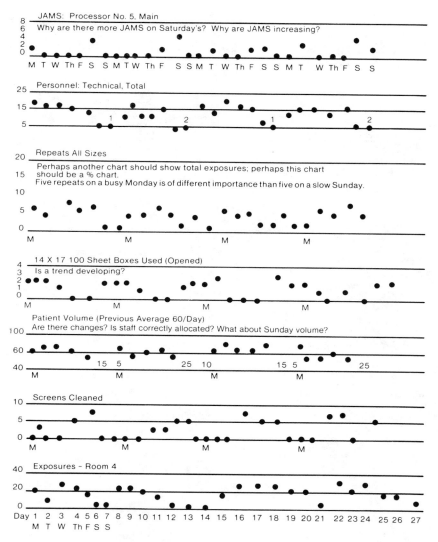

Fig. 11-54.   Other factors that could be charted.

For each processor, there are speed and contrast trend charts. These are followed by the density readings for each of 3 weeks. The mean or average for the week is determined and placed on the trend chart as an asterisk. This permits easy assessment of how the weekly averages are trending. Next the average or total mean for the month is determined. Comparing the monthly average to weekly averages should show which weeks are similar and which are dissimilar. It should also indicate which weeks are sufficiently different to pull the average toward them. The next calculation is standard deviation, which tells where 68% of the data lie ($\overline{X} \pm 1$ standard deviation) or 95% ($\overline{X}$

PROCESSOR: C1

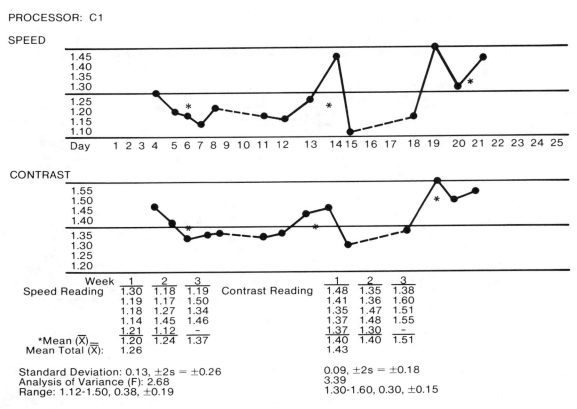

Week	1	2	3	Contrast Reading	1	2	3
Speed Reading	1.30	1.18	1.19		1.48	1.35	1.38
	1.19	1.17	1.50		1.41	1.36	1.60
	1.18	1.27	1.34		1.35	1.47	1.51
	1.14	1.45	1.46		1.37	1.48	1.55
	1.21	1.12	–		1.37	1.30	–
*Mean ($\overline{X}$)	1.20	1.24	1.37		1.40	1.40	1.51
Mean Total ($\overline{\overline{X}}$):	1.26				1.43		

Standard Deviation: 0.13, ±2s = ±0.26
Analysis of Variance (F): 2.68
Range: 1.12-1.50, 0.38, ±0.19

0.09, ±2s = ±0.18
3.39
1.30-1.60, 0.30, ±0.15

Fig. 11-55.   Statistical analysis: processor C1.

± 2s). In processor C1, for example, the weekly averages ($\overline{X}$) are 1.20, 1.24, and 1.37, with an overall average ($\overline{\overline{X}}$) of 1.26. Obviously, week 3 is pulling the average toward it. The standard deviation is 0.13, thus $\overline{X}$ + 1s and $\overline{X}$ − 1s would be 1.26 + 0.13 and 1.26 − 0.13, or 1.26 ± 0.13. Thus the trend chart should be set up with an aim or midpoint of 1.26. If we allow ±15% speed shift, then the standard deviation would fall within this range since it is only ±0.13. However, 2s (standard deviation) is usual and 3s preferred for Shewhart charts. This would be 1.26 ± 2s, or 1.26 ± 0.26. However, the trend chart scale would have to be plus 0.26 and minus 0.26 to ensure that 95% of all data falls inside the chart and ±26%, which is unacceptable. Speed acceptability is ±15% density, and contrast is ±10%. In C1, the standard deviation is too large for both speed and contrast. Thus, the process is not in control. Analysis of variance of F factor indicates the degree to which one set of data, such as 1 week, varies from another set of data. The larger the variance, the larger is the spread in sets of data. If all the data (3 weeks) overlapped, there would be a smaller value. If they virtually lined up on top of each other, there would be an extremely small value. C1, C11, C21, and C31 show four levels of variance, with C1 being high and C31 being very low. In each of these, speed and contrast are relative. In C41, speed is very high while contrast is very low. The various trend charts should indicate this. When speed and contrast track together, this is an indication of general underdevelopment. This is not necessarily a deficiency but simply means that more activity is possible from the system. Range, statistically, is expressed as zero to a maximum, but range charts are seldom used in radiography quality control. They do provide some additional insight since they show extremes. They are easy to calculate. In C1, for speed, the highest and lowest density readings form the range. Subtracting the two values produces a difference. Since ideally the average is the middle of the range and the aim or midpoint on the trend chart, it is desirable to consider this value as an arbitrary plus-and-minus value. In C1, the range of 1.12 to 1.50 is a difference of 0.38, or ±0.19. This means that all density readings lie between 1.11 and 1.51, and the midpoint in this range is 1.12 + 0.19, or 1.31 (1.50 − 0.19 = 1.31),

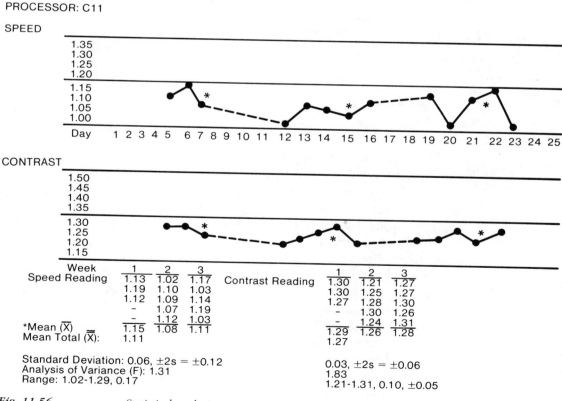

PROCESSOR: C11

SPEED

CONTRAST

Week	1	2	3		1	2	3
Speed Reading	1.13	1.02	1.17	Contrast Reading	1.30	1.21	1.27
	1.19	1.10	1.03		1.30	1.25	1.27
	1.12	1.09	1.14		1.27	1.28	1.30
	–	1.07	1.19		–	1.30	1.26
	–	1.12	1.03		–	1.24	1.31
*Mean ($\overline{X}$)	1.15	1.08	1.11		1.29	1.26	1.28
Mean Total ($\overline{\overline{X}}$):	1.11				1.27		

Standard Deviation: 0.06, ±2s = ±0.12
Analysis of Variance (F): 1.31
Range: 1.02-1.29, 0.17

0.03, ±2s = ±0.06
1.83
1.21-1.31, 0.10, ±0.05

Fig. 11-56.   Statistical analysis: processor C11.

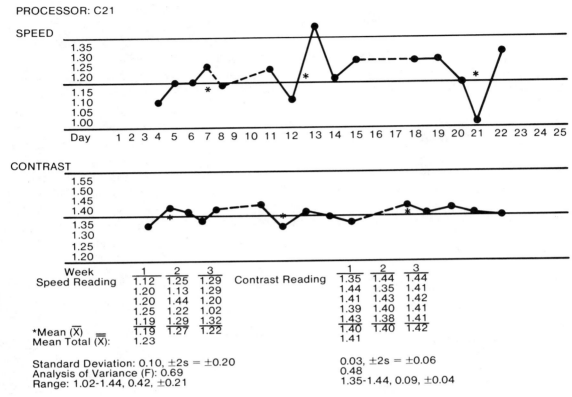

PROCESSOR: C21

Week	1	2	3		1	2	3
Speed Reading	1.12	1.25	1.29	Contrast Reading	1.35	1.44	1.44
	1.20	1.13	1.29		1.44	1.35	1.41
	1.20	1.44	1.20		1.41	1.43	1.42
	1.25	1.22	1.02		1.39	1.40	1.41
	1.19	1.29	1.32		1.43	1.38	1.41
*Mean $(\overline{X})$ =	1.19	1.27	1.22		1.40	1.40	1.42
Mean Total $(\overline{\overline{X}})$:	1.23				1.41		

Standard Deviation: 0.10, ±2s = ±0.20   0.03, ±2s = ±0.06
Analysis of Variance (F): 0.69   0.48
Range: 1.02-1.44, 0.42, ±0.21   1.35-1.44, 0.09, ±0.04

Fig. 11-57.   Statistical analysis: processor C21.

which is a little higher than the total average $(\overline{X})$ of 1.26. There are some high values that are pulling the scale upward.

Each processor is statistically analyzed for speed values and contrast values. A brief analysis follows for each, with a conclusion.

Finally, the data on the five processors were treated as a whole, and thus the entire department is evaluated for speed and contrast. The speed histogram shows a bimodal distribution on the low side, and the analysis of variance chart shows the problem to be processor C31. The other four processors are well matched, although C1 is a little on the high side. The contrast histogram shows bimodal distribution on the high side, which the variance chart indicates is C1. Notice that C1 is displaced farther from the pack for contrast than C31 is displaced for speed. This is why the contrast variance is larger. C31 was low for speed and is also low but acceptable for contrast. Thus C31 is generally underdeveloping. C1 has normal contrast but overactivity, causing excess and unacceptable speed.

In conclusion, it would appear that statistics involve a lot of additional work and provide dubious benefits. The computer program generated all of these data and more in 30 minutes. Even without the computer, using a simple calculator to derive the mean is easy and useful. Keep in mind that the primary purpose of control charts is to help the operator make decisions (the correct decision at the correct time). Statistical analysis, whether basic or complex, can aid in the trend chart interpretation, in the decision-making process. Trend chart interpretation can lead to a very reasonable and yet incorrect decision. Statistics will act as a check-and-balance system in trend chart interpretation. For example, did you notice that for processor C1 the speed aim is 1.30 but the mean is 1.26; for C21 the aim is 1.20 and the mean is 1.23. This means that C1 trend chart plots on the low side and C21 on the high side. Actually, they both should have an aim of either 1.20 or 1.25. They both have about the same standard deviation and range. The charts might suggest that C11 has a more violent swing, but certainly C21 is not stable. The analysis of variance says that the data for C1 are widely spread out while

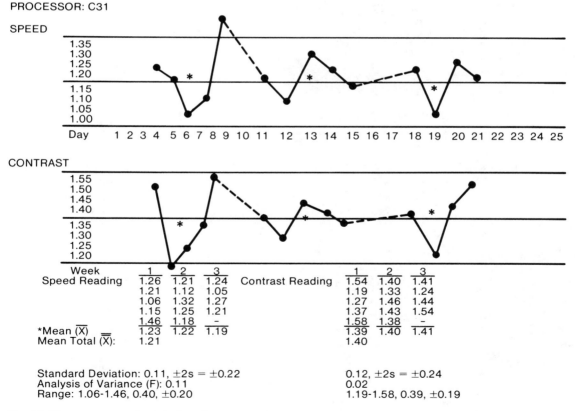

PROCESSOR: C31

Week	1	2	3	Contrast Reading	1	2	3
Speed Reading	1.26	1.21	1.24		1.54	1.40	1.41
	1.21	1.12	1.05		1.19	1.33	1.24
	1.06	1.32	1.27		1.27	1.46	1.44
	1.15	1.25	1.21		1.37	1.43	1.54
	1.46	1.18	–		1.58	1.38	–
*Mean (X̄)	1.23	1.22	1.19		1.39	1.40	1.41
Mean Total (X̿):	1.21				1.40		

Standard Deviation: 0.11, ±2s = ±0.22   0.12, ±2s = ±0.24
Analysis of Variance (F): 0.11   0.02
Range: 1.06-1.46, 0.40, ±0.20   1.19-1.58, 0.39, ±0.19

Fig. 11-58.   Statistical analysis: processor C31.

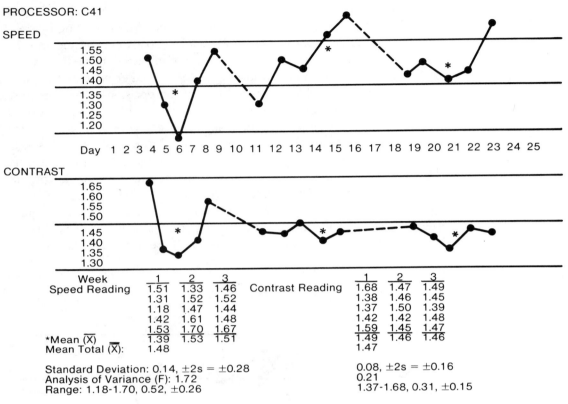

PROCESSOR: C41

Week	1	2	3		Contrast Reading	1	2	3
Speed Reading	1.51	1.33	1.46			1.68	1.47	1.49
	1.31	1.52	1.52			1.38	1.46	1.45
	1.18	1.47	1.44			1.37	1.50	1.39
	1.42	1.61	1.48			1.42	1.42	1.48
	1.53	1.70	1.67			1.59	1.45	1.47
*Mean (X̄)	1.39	1.53	1.51			1.49	1.46	1.46
Mean Total (X̄):	1.48					1.47		

Standard Deviation: 0.14, ±2s = ±0.28   0.08, ±2s = ±0.16
Analysis of Variance (F): 1.72   0.21
Range: 1.18-1.70, 0.52, ±0.26   1.37-1.68, 0.31, ±0.15

Fig. 11-59.   Statistical analysis: processor C41.

for C21 they are generally excellent. Obviously, what we see as charts or pictures is interpreted somewhat subjectively, whereas numbers offer objectivity. Note that the trend chart in C1 has an aim of 1.30 and the scale is ±0.20. The actual data ranged ±0.19, with an average of 1.26. This is very good correlation. However, based on an average of 1.26 and a standard deviation of 0.13, ±2s indicates that if we want 95% of the data to be inside the chart's limits then the chart would be set up as 1.26 ± 0.26, or 1.00 − 1.52. This approximates a ±26% speed density change and is much too broad, thus the system is out of control. If the speed is in control, then the 2s or even 3s level should be within ±0.15 density units from the midpoint.

Analysis of Processor C1

- In Figure 11-55, speed is averaging 1.26 ± 0.13; analysis of variance suggests there is an upward trend. The histogram is bimodal at the high end. A problem is beginning. This agrees with the trend chart. The range is excessive.
- Contrast averages 1.40 and has a small standard deviation of 0.09 but a

high variance, indicating a problem. The histogram is bimodal at the high end (week 3). Again this confirms trend chart indication of trend to higher levels. Range is excessive.

- Adjust the replenishment rate lower, or lower developer temperature. Confirm speed.

Analysis of Processor C11

- In Figure 11-56, speed is averaging 1.11, which is low. Variance is not too high, suggesting consistency.
- Contrast is very stable but is probably low.

Compared with C1 and C21, this processor is in control but generally underdeveloping. Raise the replenishment rate after starting over with fresh chemicals. If fresh chemicals do not raise activity, then the replenishment rate is probably satisfactory. Raise the temperature 2°F (15%).

Analysis of Processor C21

- In Figure 11-57, speed appears to have an acceptable average. Variance is very low, indicating consistency. The range is too large because of days 13 and 21.
- Contrast is extremely stable.
- Speed changes on days 13 and 21 are probably temperature fluctuations (assignable cause), since the process remains in control the rest of the time.

Analysis of Processor C31

- In Figure 11-58, speed is consistent except for day 8, which causes the large range. Variance is very small. The histogram is bimodal at the low end.
- Contrast is stable, although it has many swings. Variance is not a good indicator because of the large range in each week and overall. The histogram shows normal distribution.
- The trend charts show contrast and speed tracking together, indicating an underdevelopment situation.

Analysis of Processor C41

- In Figure 11-59, speed has a high average, with last 2 weeks about equal. The histogram shows normal distribution but very wide; the range is excessively large, suggesting that the process is out of control.
- Contrast is more stable and in control. Variance is small. Range deviation would be smaller if day 4 were eliminated.
- Something is affecting speed. It is probably an unassigned variable such as contamination.

Analysis of Combined Speed

- The histogram shows bimodal distribution, indicating a problem (Fig. 11-60).
- Analysis of variance (F) is very large, indicating a problem. The chart shows C1 to have an abnormally high mean, whereas the other four processors are matched. C1 does not overlap any other processors. C31 overlaps three processors, indicating similarity, although it is on the low side.

PROCESSOR: All (C1, C11, C21, C31, C41)

COMBINED SPEED

Processor:	C1	C11	C21	C31	C41
Mean ($\overline{X}$):	1.46	1.25	1.24	1.22	1.25

Total Mean($\overline{\overline{X}}$): 1.26
Std. Deviation: 0.16, $\pm 2s = \pm 0.32$
Anal. Variance (F): 14.40

Range: 1.02-1.70
ΔR: 0.68
$\pm$: 0.34

Observations: Histogram

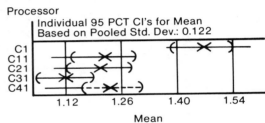

Fig. 11-60.   Statistical analysis: departmental speed.

PROCESSOR: All (C1, C11, C21, C31, C41)

COMBINED CONTRAST

Processor:	C1	C11	C21	C31	C41
Mean ($\overline{X}$):	1.47	1.39	1.42	1.29	1.42

Total Mean ($\overline{\overline{X}}$): 1.40
Std. Deviation: 0.10, $\pm 2s = \pm 0.20$
Anal. Variance (F): 9.38

Range: 1.19-1.68
ΔR: 0.49
$\pm$: 0.25

Observations: Histogram

Fig. 11-61.   Statistical analysis: departmental contrast.

Analysis of Combined Contrast

- The histogram shows an approximately normal distribution with a slight trend toward bimodal at the lower end, suggesting a marginally out-of-control process (Fig. 11-61).
- The analysis of variance (F) is very large, indicating a problem. The chart shows that C31 is beyond the range of the other processors and is abnormally but only marginally low, since lines almost overlap.

Analysis of All Processors for July, 1983

- Speed is an average of 1.26; charts should be set with an aim or midpoint of D 1.20. Processor C1 is too active by approximately 20%. The other processors are matched and in control.
- Contrast is an average of 1.40; charts should be set with an aim or midpoint of 1.40. Processor C31 is exhibiting low contrast and slightly low speed, suggesting that a minor change in activity or temperature will correct the process. The other four processors are matched in control. Note that C1 is slightly high in contrast and very high in speed, suggesting a need to lower the activity.

Appendix I

Suggested Reading List/Bibliography

Very few texts or research papers deal specifically with radiographic processing, since radiography is a specialized area of photographic science. All of the references listed below contain useful sections that will help increase one's understanding of the importance, function, and problematic areas of radiographic processing. Recommended primary sources are indicated by a bullet (•).

Reference Texts

- • *The Theory of the Photographic Process,* 3rd ed. By C.E.K. Mees and T.H. James. Macmillian, NY, 1971.

  The Theory of the Photographic Process. By C.E.K. Mees. Macmillian, NY, 1954.

  Fundamentals of Photographic Theory. By T.H. James and G.C. Higgins. Morgan and Morgan, NY, 1960.

  Fundamental Mechanisms of Photographic Sensitivity. Edited by J.W. Mitchell. Butterworth & Co, London, 1951.

  The Physics of Medical Imaging. Edited by A. Haus, American Institute of Physics, 335 East 45th St., NY 10017. Papers from the 1979 Summer School of the American Association of Physicists in Medicine, 1979.

The Photographic Action of Ionizing Radiation. By R.H. Herz, John Wiley & Sons, NY, 1969.

Photographic Processing, Quality Control and the Evaluation of Photographic Materials, Vols. I and II. By J.E. Gray. HEW Publication (FDA) 77-8018 (Bureau of Radiologer Health, Rockville, MD) Vol. II lists references and resources and is particularly useful.

• *Radiographic Processing and Film Quality Control.* By W. E. J. McKinney for the U.S. Veterans Administration, Radiological Services. This is a set of 16 half-hour videotapes on radiographic processing including electromechanical systems, image formation, history, chemistry, artifacts, sensitometry, and quality control. Available from the VA learning centers, the American Society of Radiologic Technologists, or from the Du Pont Company. Customer Technology Center, Wilmington, DE 19898.

• *Radiographic Processing and Film Quality Control.* By C.C. Kirby, T.T. Thompson, and W.E.J. McKinney. American Society of Radiologic Technologists, 1975. This guide reviews and supplements the tape series listed above but may be used separately.

Darkroom Technique Guide. E.I. Du Pont de Nemours & Company, Wilmington, DE, 1960.

• *Photographic Sensitometry.* By H.N. Todd and R.D. Zakia. Morgan and Morgan, NY, 1969.

Photographic Sensitometry: A Self Teaching Text. By H.N. Todd. John Wiley & Sons, NY, 1977.

Sensitometric Properties of X-Ray Film. Eastman Kodak. Rochester, NY, 1963.

• *Photographic Processing Chemistry.* By L.F.A. Mason, Focal Library, NY, 1975.

• *Modern Photographic Processing.* By G. Haist. 200 volumes. John Wiley & Sons, NY, 1978.

Control Techniques in Film Processing. Society of Motion Picture and Television Engineers (SMPTE), 19606 East 41st St., NY 10017.

Handbook of Photography, Society of Photographic Scientists and Engineers (SPSE). Suite 204, 1330 Massachusetts Ave., NW, Washington, DC 20005.

* *Principles of Chemistry.* By D.C. Gregg. Allyn and Bacon, Boston, 1963.

* *College Chemistry.* By L. Pauling. Freeman, San Francisco, 1964.
  Applied Processing Practice and Technics. Edited by R.H. Gray. Society of Photographic Scientists and Engineers (SPSE), Washington, DC, 1968.

* *Basic Electricity.* By A. Marcus, Prentice-Hall, Englewood Cliffs, 1958.

* *Bit System of Technic Conversion,* 8th ed. By R.J. Trinkle. E.I. Du Pont de Nemours & Co, Wilmington, DE, 1982.

* *Introduction to Electronics. I.* By B. Grob. McGraw-Hill, NY, 1959.

* *Your Guide to Photography.* By H.F. Bruce, Barnes and Noble, NY.

* *Photography.* By P. Hillson. Doubleday Science Series, NY.

* *Basic Chemistry of Photographic Processing,* Parts 1 and 2. Eastman Kodak, Rochester, NY. These are self-teaching texts.

* These are representative texts. Any similar text will substitute and serve the purpose.

Caboon's Formulating X-Ray Technics, 9th ed. By T.T. Thompson. Duke University Press, Durham, NC, 1979.

- *Quality Assurance in Diagnostic Radiology.* By J.M. McLemore. Year Book Medical Publishers, Chicago, 1981.

Silver Recovery. E.I. Du Pont de Nemours & Co., Wilmington, DE.

Dollars and Cents of Silver Recovery. E.I. Du Pont de Nemours & Co., Wilmington, DE.

Acceptance Testing of Radiological Imaging Equipment. Edited by P.P. Lin. AAPM Monograph of Seminar Proceedings, AAPM, 1981.

How to Manage Your Silver Recovery System to Meet Silver Discharge Regulations, Vol.1, No.1. IMG Photo Products, 1733 Rogers Avenue, San Jose, CA 95112-1184, 1986.

Statistics. By J.T. McClave and F.H. Dietrich, III. Dellen Publishing Co., San Francisco, 1979.

Statistical Quality Control Methods. By I.W. Burr. Vol. 16 of *Statistics: Textbooks and Monographs.* Edited by D.B. Owen. Marcel Dekker, NY, 1976.

Quality Assurance, Management & Technology, 5th ed. By G.E. Hayes. Charger Productions, Capistrano, 1982.

Quality is Free. By P.B. Crosby. McGraw-Hill, NY, 1979.

Quality Control Handbook, 3rd ed. By J.M. Juron. McGraw Hill, NY, 1979.

Quality Control in Diagnostic Imaging. By J.E. Gray, N.T. Winkler, et al., University Park Press, Baltimore, 1983.

Radiographic Latent Image Processing, Sec. 7, "The Nondestructive Testing Handbook on Radiography and Radiation Testing." By W.E.J. McKinney. ASNT, Columbus, OH, 1982.

Reference Journals and Proceedings

Journal of Photographic Engineering
Journal of Photographic Society of America
Journal of Colloid Science
Journal of Physical Chemistry
Journal of the Society of Motion Picture and Television Engineers (SMPTE)
Journal of the Society of Photographic Scientists and Engineers (SPSE)
National Electric Code by Fire Underwriters Association, available from local underwriters

Technical Magazines

American Photographer
Photographic Science and Technology
Photographic Scientific Engineering
Scientific Industrial Photography

Industrial Photography
Radiography
Photo Methods for Industry
Technical Photography
Photographic Science and Engineering
Quality Control by the American Society for Quality Control, Chicago
Physics Today

Appendix II

Quiz

1. Describe how to test safelights properly.
2. Are films safe under safelights? Explain your answer.
3. List the basic safelight conditions: lamp wattage _____ distance to film _____
4. The darkroom should be painted what color?
5. The tops of processors provide additional counter space. T or F
6. Describe how to test view-box quality.
7. Light rooms should be as bright as possible. T or F
8. Film and chemicals should be stored at _____°C (_____°F) or less and _____% RH.
9. Cassettes and screens should be cleaned _____ (how often) and checked radiographically _____ (how often).
10. Film base is made from
    a. polyethylene
    b. cellulose acetate
    c. cellulose triacetate
    d. polyethylene terephalate
11. Emulsions are really suspensions. T or F

12. Emulsions are composed of which of the following:
    a. Binder   d. Silver halide salts
    b. Gelatin   e. Silver bromides
    c. Tint   f. Recording media
13. Define sensitometry.
14. Define density in a clinical sense and in a technical sense.
15. A logarithm is a number system based on powers of 10. T or F
16. List four measurable sensitometric values
    (1) _____   (3) _____
    (2) _____   (4) _____
17. How do D_{min} and B+F differ?
18. What are the three components of B+F?
19. Give examples of the following:
    Indicated speed
    Calculated speed
    Indicated contrast
    Calculated contrast
20. Contrast measurements are based on
    a. the gamma of the straight-line portion
    b. a gradient point based on a density or exposure point on the
       H&D curve
    c. the average slope between coordinates 2.00 + B+F and
       0.25 + B+F
    d. all of the above
21. What is the difference between manual and automatic processing?
22. What is unique about automatic developers?
23. Gurney-Mott developed the modern bellows replenishment
    pump. T or F
24. What is the function of the developer?
25. Oxidation produces _____; reduction uses _____.
26. In forming the visible image, the developer is _____ and the
    exposed silver halide crystals are reduced to _____.
27. List three ways in which the developer can be oxidized or
    consumed.
    (1) _____   (2) _____   (3) _____
28. What elements control all chemical reactions?
29. Activity is very important when considering time/temperature
    relationship. Why?
30. How is the time factor defined and measured?
31. Starter is used to activate or start up the developer. T or F
32. Name six processor systems that support the needs of the
    chemical system:
    (1) _____   (2) _____   (3) _____
    (4) _____   (5) _____   (6) _____

33. Which of the seven systems is the source of most problems?
34. How much stronger is a pH of 2 than a pH of 3?
35. Specific gravity of a film should be a density of 0.20. T or F
36. The density of developer when measured with a hydrometer is heavier than water. T or F
37. When chemicals are measured for pH or specific gravity, the _____ must be adjusted for because it influences and controls activity of the chemicals.
38. Hydroquinone controls what part of the H&D curve?
39. Phenidone is hyperactive to temperature rise and causes chemical _____.
40. Superadditivity results from _____.
41. Are developers generally acid or alkaline?
42. The preservative keeps the developer from coagulating like jelly. T or F
43. The solvent for developer and fixer is any petroleum solvent. T or F
44. Should the mixing of developer be vigorous or mild, just enough, or prolonged?
45. The developer is hazardous, but the fixer is more so. T or F
46. Explain how fixer fixes the film.
47. What are the three functions of the fixer?
    (1) _____ (2) _____ (3) _____
48. What is the weakest component of all the chemicals components that often leads to fixer and wash problems?
49. Which of the following is not associated with fixer?
    a. Clearing
    b. fixing
    c. Hypo
    d. Glutaraldehyde
    e. Sodium sulfite
50. Describe a clearing time-test procedure in two steps.
    (1) _____ (2) _____
51. What is the chemical function of the water?
52. The mechanical function of the water is to
    a. wash the tank
    b. wash the film
    c. help control developer temperature
    d. improve archival quality
    e. agitate the solution
53. Define archival quality.
54. List two methods of determining the archival quality of a film.
    (1) _____ (2) _____

55. What are four factors that can contribute to poor archival quality?
    (1) _____ (2) _____
    (3) _____ (4) _____
56. Storage conditions for archival-quality film must be at least 25°C (77°F) and a 75% RH. T or F
57. The transport system controls what function?
58. Temperature control is influenced by processor location. T or F
59. List four functions of the circulation/filtration system:
    (1) _____ (2) _____
    (3) _____ (4) _____
60. Define the difference between a thermometer and a thermostat.
61. Thermometers may be calibrated and should be tested for accuracy about once a year. T or F. What's wrong with this statement?
62. Mixing valves are failsafe to hot mechanisms, which means that they turn on hot water if the heater fails. T or F
63. Pumps are composed of three parts:
    (1) _____ (2) _____ (3) _____
64. Define replenishment of chemicals.
    Define regeneration of chemicals.
65. List five causes of noninformational density.
    (1) _____ (2) _____ (3) _____
    (4) _____ (5) _____
66. What is head pressure variation?
67. Dryers become more efficient toward the end of the day. T, F, or maybe.
68. Clean dryer rollers influence drying efficiency. T or F
69. Wet film may be caused by failed or inefficient dryer _____ even if the heaters and blowers are okay.
70. What are three general areas used in progressive quality control?
    (1) _____ (2) _____ (3) _____
71. Why is sensitometry the single best tool for measuring quality control?
72. Sensitometric quality control is a procedure to develop better quality. T or F
73. Artifacts are
    a. made by hand
    b. defects
    c. plus density
    d. minus density
    e. physical damage
    f. all of the above

74. List two main areas where artifacts may be produced in addition to darkroom/handling.

    (1) _____ (2) _____

75. List three different light sources for viewing films—especially artifacts.

    (1) _____ (2) _____ (3) _____

76. List four common clues on most films.

    (1) _____ (2) _____

    (3) _____ (4) _____

77. What causes dichroic stain?

78. Curtain effect may be on either the leading edge or the trailing edge of the film and is further called, respectively, _____ and

    _____ .

79. List two ways of telling film direction through a processor.

    (1) _____ (2) _____

80. In all photography, what is unique about x-ray film that must be remembered when trying to determine the cause of artifacts?

81. Silver recovery is most important because it returns most of the cost of the film to the department. T or F

82. The most common method of silver recovery is precipitation. T or F

83. Scrap film is sold by the pound, and more money is made by selling it a pound at a time. T or F

84. Electrolytic units are called cells because they

    a. have bars like a jail

    b. trap silver and hold it like a jail

    c. are square

    d. are constructed like a battery

85. A terminal recovery unit is one that is worn out and ready to be replaced. T or F

86. What are the anatomic parts of the H&D curve?

87. H&D stands for higher and deeper, as the density response is plotted against the exposure stimulus. T or F

88. Security of film is economically much more important than silver recovery. On a scale of 1 to 10, how much more important? 1, 2, 3, 4, 5, 6, 7, 8, 9, 10

89. In the transport system, sprockets and gears have numbers that allow them to be matched together. T or F

90. Static is most often produced by an ungrounded processor feed tray. T or F

91. The developer amplifies the latent image into the visible image by a factor of 10^2, or 100 times. T or F

92. Floating lids on replenishment tanks control developer _____ and fixer _____.
93. How is the correct replenishment rate for developer determined?
94. As above, for fixer?
95. If the hydroquinone fails, what happens to the H&D curve?
96. If anything fails in the photographic system, it is usually seen as a loss of contrast. T or F
97. View boxes can influence contrast. T or F
98. Processing completes what the exposure started. T or F
99. Antifoggants are also called restrainers because _____.
100. When feeding a film into a processor, flip the film toward the slot to avoid placing fingers on the surface. T or F

Answers

1. Preexpose film, place under light, turn on, and expose strips at 10-second intervals.
2. No, unless tested. Even then there will be a time limit.
3. $7\frac{1}{2}$ to 15   121 cm (4 ft)
4. Any light color
5. F
6. With a light meter, measure the exposure value (EV) at ASA 100.
7. F
8. 21°C   (70°F)   40 to 60% RH
9. Weekly, quarterly
10. d
11. T
12. a, b, d, e, f,
13. Quantitative measure of the film's response to exposure and development
14. Amount of blackness or silver on or in film; logarithm of inverse of transmittance, LOG 1/T or LOG $\dfrac{1}{I_0/I_1}$ or LOG $\dfrac{I_1}{I_0}$
15. T
16. D_{min}, D_{max}, speed, contrast
17. D_{min} is the minimum density for the minimum exposure. B + F is inherent.
18. Base density, tint density, fog density
19. Reading the density of step on the gray scale closest to 1.00.

    Calculate based on the energy needed to produce a density of 1.00 + B + F on H&D curve.

* Read the density of two steps on the gray scale and subtract the smaller from the larger.

   Measure the slope of the angle on the H&D curve between coordinates 2.00 + B+F and 0.25 + B+F.
20. d
21. Manual processing has human controls.
22. They have a hardener.
23. F
24. To convert the latent image into the visible image
25. Electrons, electrons
26. Oxidized, metallic silver
27. Silver development, aerial, contamination
28. Time/temperature/activity
29. Without controlled activity, the time/temperature relationship won't work.
30. As immersion time in solution: leading edge of a film into solution until leading edge out of the solution
31. F
32. Transport, temperature, circulation/filtration, regeneration/replenishment, electrical, and dryer
33. Chemistry
34. 10 times, or 100%
35. F
36. T
37. Temperature
38. Shoulder
39. Fog
40. The interaction of hydroquinone and phenidone
41. Alkaline
42. F
43. F
44. Mild, just enough
45. F
46. Prevents further exposure, development, and prepares for drying and storage
47. Stop or neutralize the developer, clear away all remaining silver halide crystals, shrink and harden the emulsion
48. Glutaraldehyde (developer hardener)
49. d
50. Clear a green strip. Dip second patch, and time until clear to match first patch.
51. Dilute out fixer.
52. c

53. Remaining unchanged for a period of time
54. Estimator kits, submit a film to film company for ANSI procedure
55. Developer hardener, fixer activity, washing, storage
56. F
57. Time
58. T
59. Mix for uniform temperature, uniform activity, filtration, agitation
60. Thermometer indicates (measures, reads); a thermostat regulates.
61. F (weekly)
62. F
63. Motor, coupler, pump head
64. Sustain volume or levels; sustain activity
65. Overexposure, light, heat, radiation, overdevelopment (temperature, replenish) static, pressure, age, contamination
66. Changes in height of fluid in replenishment tank
67. Maybe
68. T
69. Exhaust
70. Electromechanical, chemical, sensitometric
71. Measures total effect and is the product produced.
72. F
73. f
74. Exposure, processing
75. Transmitted, reflected, bright
76. Date, guide shoe marks, film stencil, screen stencil, nonscreen area
77. Chemical failure
78. Runback, rundown
79. Guide shoe marks, pi marks, moisture streaks
80. Two emulsion layers (sides)
81. F
82. F
83. F
84. d
85. F
86. Toe, shoulder, straight-line portion (body)
87. F
88. 10
89. F
90. F
91. F
92. Oxidation, fumes
93. Bromide level
94. Silver level

95. The shoulder falls
96. T
97. T
98. T
99. They restrain the reducing agents from producing chemical fog.
100. F

Index

Numbers followed by *f* indicate figures.